Enteral and Pare

A CLINICAL HANDBOOK

EDITED BY

ANDREW GRANT
MB, ChB, MRCP, D.Phil
Lecturer in Chemical Pathology
Department of
Chemical Pathology
Old Medical School
Leeds LS2 9JT

ELIZABETH TODD
BSc, SRD
Formerly Chief Dietitian
Department of
Nutrition and Dietetics
John Radcliffe Hospital
Oxford OX3 9DU

Nursing Adviser
SUSAN ATKINS
RGN, SCM, DN, RNT
Nurse Tutor
John Radcliffe Hospital
Oxford OX3 9DU

SECOND EDITION

Blackwell Scientific Publications
OXFORD LONDON EDINBURGH
BOSTON PALO ALTO MELBOURNE

© 1982, 1987 by
Blackwell Scientific Publications
Editorial offices:
Osney Mead, Oxford OX2 0EL
  (*Orders*: Tel. 0865 240201)
8 John Street, London WC1N 2ES
23 Ainslie Place, Edinburgh EH3 6AJ
52 Beacon Street, Boston
  Massachusetts 02108, USA
667 Lytton Avenue, Palo Alto
  California 94301, USA
107 Barry Street, Carlton
  Victoria 3053, Australia

First published 1982
Second edition 1987

Set by Colset Private Ltd
Singapore
Printed and bound
in Great Britain

DISTRIBUTORS

USA
  Year Book Medical Publishers
  35 East Wacker Drive
  Chicago, Illinois 60601
  (*Orders*: Tel. 312 726-9733)

Canada
  The C.V. Mosby Company
  5240 Finch Avenue East,
  Scarborough, Ontario
  (*Orders*: Tel. 416-298-1588)

Australia
  Blackwell Scientific Publications
  (Australia) Pty Ltd
  107 Barry Street
  Carlton, Victoria 3053
  (*Orders*: Tel. (03) 347 0300)

British Library
Cataloguing in Publication Data

Enteral and parenteral nutrition: a
  clinical handbook. — 2nd ed.
  1. Parenteral feeding
  I. Grant, Andrew   II. Todd,
  Elizabeth
  615.8'54   RM224

  ISBN 0-632-01786-4

Contents

Contents

Contributors

Susan Atkins RGN, SCM, DN RNT *Nurse Tutor, John Radcliffe Hospital, Oxford OX3 9DU*

John F Burke MD, FACS *Professor of Surgery, Harvard Medical School, Chief of Trauma, Massachusetts General Hospital, Boston, Massachusetts, USA*

Helen Chapel MA, MD, MRCPath *Department of Immunopathology, John Radcliffe Hospital, Oxford OX3 9DU*

Paul Collinson MB, MRCPath *Senior Registrar, Department of Chemical Pathology and Human Metabolism, Royal Free Hospital, London NW3 2QG*

Ashley Dennison MB, ChB, FRCS *Senior Registrar, Department of Surgery, Nottingham City Hospital, Hucknall Road, Nottingham NG5 1PB*

Andrew Grant MB, ChB, MRCP, DPhil *Lecturer and Consultant in Chemical Pathology, Department of Chemical Pathology, Old Medical School, Leeds LS2 9JT*

Michael Greenall BSc, MB, ChB, FRCS, FRCS(Ed) *Consultant Surgeon, John Radcliffe Hospital, Oxford OX3 9DU*

Linda Hands MBBS, FRCS *Research Fellow, Nuffield Department of Surgery, John Radcliffe Hospital, Oxford OX3 9DU*

Peter Harper MCh, FRCS *Senior Registrar, Department of Surgery, Royal Victoria Infirmary, Newcastle upon Tyne NE1 4LP*

Richard Jones MD, MRCP *Senior Registrar, Department of Chemical Pathology, Old Medical School, Leeds LS2 9JT*

Hugh Kennedy MD, MRCP *Consultant Physician, Norfolk and Norwich Hospital, Norwich, Norfolk*

Michael Kettlewell MA, MB, MC, FRCS *Consultant Surgeon, John Radcliffe Hospital, Oxford OX3 9DU*

Michael J. McMahon ChM, PhD, FRCS *Senior Lecturer/Consultant Surgeon PhD University Department of Surgery, The General Infirmary, Leeds LS1 3EX*

Andrew Mitchell MCh, FRCS *Consultant Surgeon, Milton Keynes General Hospital, Milton Keynes MK6 5LD*

Tony Nunn B Pharm MPS *Principal Pharmacist, Alder Hey Children's Hospital, Eaton Road, Liverpool L12 2AP*

Stephen O'Keefe MD, MSc, MRCP *Consultant Physician, Groote Schuur Hospital, University of Capetown, South Africa*

L Rangecroft FRCS *Consultant Paediatric Surgeon, Newcastle Hospital for Sick Children, Great North Road, Newcastle upon Tyne NE2 3AX*

Karen Ross SRD *Paediatric Dietitian, John Radcliffe Hospital, Oxford OX3 9DU*

Gavin Royle MS, FRCS *Senior Lecturer, Department of Surgery, Southampton University, Southampton SO9 5NH*

Christopher Taylor MD, MRCP, DCH *Senior Lecturer in Child Health, Alder Hey Children's Hospital, Eaton Road, Liverpool L12 2AP*

Elizabeth Todd BSc, SRD *Formerly Senior Dietitian, John Radcliffe Hospital, Oxford OX3 9DU*

Christopher Winearls MB, DPhil, MRCP *Senior Registrar, Renal Unit, Hammersmith Hospital, London W12 0HS*

Bryan Winsley PhD, FPS *Principal Pharmacist, John Radcliffe Hospital, Oxford OX3 9DU*

Preface to the Second Edition

An increased awareness of the nutritional needs of the patient is occurring in British hospital practice, but it cannot be said that the spectre of nutritional neglect has been eliminated. The team approach has proved invaluable with co-operation between doctor, nurse, pharmacist, dietitian and biochemist.

In this second edition, which has been expanded to include paediatrics, we continue to apply a broad approach to the nutritional therapy of the vulnerable patient and enourage the reader to view parenteral nutrition within the full range of feeding possibilities.

We would like to thank the many people who have supported our efforts and especially the secretarial help of Tracey Turner and her team.

Oxford   Andrew Grant
                                                     Elizabeth Todd

Preface to the First Edition

The recognition that nutritional neglect can occur in modern hospital practice led recently to the establishment of a 'nutrition team' in several centres. The formation of the Oxford team has enabled an evaluation and improvement of feeding techniques to be carried out and has developed an invaluable co-operation between doctor, nurse, pharmacist, dietitian and biochemist.

In this book we apply a broad approach to the nutritional therapy of the vulnerable patient—whether it be extra slices of bread and butter, or total parenteral nutrition.

We wish to promote an increased awareness of the nutritional care of all patients and encourage the reader to view parenteral nutrition within the full range of feeding possibilities.

We would like to thank the many people who have supported our efforts and especially the secretarial help of Clare Flanagan, Madeline Carvell, Joanna Eadle and Doreen Hagar.

Oxford
Andrew Grant
Elizabeth Todd

Chapter 1 · Meeting Patients' Needs

The close association between malnutrition and morbidity and even mortality has been known for a long time. Recent surveys have drawn attention to unacceptable malnutrition in British (Hill *et al.* 1977; Todd *et al.* 1984) and American hospitals (Bistrian *et al.* 1974). Not only is malnutrition quite common but it is more prevalent in surgical wards, and is more severe with increasing hospital stay.

Parenteral nutrition has become a popular but probably misused treatment. It is therefore very important for clinicians and nurses to recognize those patients who should receive special nutritional support and to be able to decide rationally what form this support should take.

The clinician, dietitian or nurse needs to assess carefully the diet of any patient likely to need support, and to repeat the exercise regularly. This is in essence a return to the values of Florence Nightingale (1859) who wrote, 'Every careful observer of the sick will agree in this, that thousands of patients are annually starved in the midst of plenty, for want of attention to the ways which alone make it possible for them to take food . . . I would say to the nurse have a rule of thought about your patient's diet. Consider. Remember how much he has had and how much he ought to have today.'

Effective nutritional support can be given in several different ways. Table 1.1, p. 2, illustrates the range of support, from simple to complex. For example the appropriate means to meet the nutritional needs of an elderly patient who cannot take meals normally may simply be additional nursing care to ensure that meals are appetizing, and contain sufficient protein, calories and other nutrients. The other end of the spectrum is the patient requiring large amounts of intravenous protein and calories because of major injury.

Table 1.1. Examples to illustrate the range of nutritional support.

Methods requiring patient co-operation

Nursing support
Encouragement and help with feeding
Ensure food is eaten
Anticipation of patient's needs

Diet modification—consultation with dietitian
Special needs e.g. high calorie
Altered consistency—semi solid or liquid

Methods less dependent on active patient co-operation

Tube feeding
Nasoenteric tubes
Feeding gastrostomy
Feeding jejunostomy

If the function of the gastrointestinal tract is impaired or inadequate

Intravenous feeding
Intravenous feeding combined with enteral feeding
Peripheral vein feeding
Central vein feeding

It is the purpose of this chapter to fit the nutritional support to the individual patient. It is not easy to classify those conditions that most often require additional nutritional support. Table 1.2 gives a basic classification but clearly the support required depends on the individual patient and the extent of his disease. Assessment of the patient involves a consideration of:

1 dietary history
2 present nutritional status
3 an estimate of present and predicted needs.

DIETARY HISTORY

The dietary assessment should be considered in two parts and *recorded*. Firstly, an estimate is made of the food intake over the past few weeks by careful questioning about meal patterns, types and quantities of food normally eaten throughout the day; whether snacks or sweets are eaten between meals; whether the

Table 1.2. Examples of conditions that may require additional nutritional support.

Depressed appetite
Cancer patients—especially during chemotherapy or radiotherapy
Anorexic patients
Some chronic conditions e.g.
  renal disease
  chronic heart disease

Inability to feed
Old people living alone
Disorientation
Strokes
Coma

Gastrointestinal failure
Oesophageal obstruction e.g. stricture or cancer
Malabsorption e.g. Crohn's disease; radiation enteritis
Chronic liver disease
Pancreatitis
Protein losing enteropathy

Increased needs
Severe burns
Septicaemia
Major trauma
Excessive loss from fistulae and drains

appetite has changed recently and whether meals are eaten in company (Beal 1967).

This form of questioning will place the majority of patients into low, normal or high food intake groups (Black 1981) and so allow a reasonable judgement about the influence of diet upon a patient's current clinical state.

Secondly, an estimate should be made of a patient's intake in hospital. This allows early recognition of patients who need additional nutritional support and what form it should take. Protein and calorie values of common foods are given in the appendix pp. 259–61.

ASSESSMENT OF NUTRITIONAL STATUS

The patient's nutritional needs are in part governed by the loss of reserves at the time of presentation. Numerous means of assessing body deficit have been described and are used to guide people in the nutritional care of patients, but no clear advantage has been shown for using any of the more simple quantitative measurements or even several different ones together.

Probably the most important assessment is the clinical impression based upon the patient's history, his disease, and their effect upon body weight. This is an impression supported by such things as the feel of the subcutaneous tissues, the power in the limbs and the condition of the hair. In the hands of a sensitive clinician, the sum of these features is probably far more subtle and accurate than dependence upon numeric values for several tests whose value is doubtful (Collins *et al.* 1979; Forse & Shizgal 1980; Michel *et al.* 1981). However it is necessary to discuss some of the measurements more commonly used.

Body weight

Loss of weight is mainly made up of lost muscle, fat and fluid. Theoretically it is important to know which body compartment has suffered most because loss of lean body mass is associated with an increased wound infection rate (Cruse & Foord 1973), poor wound healing (Irvin & Hunt 1974) and possibly pulmonary complications because of reduced ventilatory capacity (Dockel *et al.* 1976). Injury and illness is usually accompanied by a loss of lean body mass. On the other hand loss of fat is of little significance in most Western people.

Actual body weight can be compared either to the optimal body weight for height, build and sex (tabulated in the appendix, pp. 218–19), or to the patient's usual or remembered body weight, and expressed as a percentage weight loss. Loss of about 10% of body weight represents mild malnutrition, moderate malnutrition 20% weight loss and severe malnutrition greater than 30% weight loss.

Peripheral oedema or dehydration lead to misinterpretation of the observed weight loss. Again, weight loss estimated from ideal body weight in obese patients can hide significant malnutrition. These caveats serve to emphasize the need to use common sense in the interpretation of weight loss. In addition, the more rapid the weight loss the more severe the malnutrition is likely to be and greater is the risk to the patient.

Anthropometric measurements

Simple measurements to assess lean body mass and fat have been described. They have proved useful in field surveys of malnutrition (Jelliffe 1966) but have not had satisfactory validation in hospital patients. The potential for observer error is great.

Skinfold thickness

Measurements of the skinfold thickness over the triceps, biceps, scapula and superior iliac crests using calipers gives an estimate of the body's subcutaneous fat reserve (Durnin & Rahaman 1967).

Triceps skinfold thickness alone has also been used to estimate fat reserve and nomograms are available (Frisancho 1974).

Mid-arm circumference

Arm circumference (AC) and triceps skinfold thickness (TST) allows arm muscle circumference (AMC) to be calculated.

$$AMC = AC - \pi TST$$

Percentile charts have been derived to be used as an index of malnutrition (Frisancho 1974; Gurney & Jelliffe 1973).

Muscle function

Muscle function is an important index of muscle mass and its integrity. Tests of respiratory function such as forced inspiratory and expiratory pressure as well as FEV (forced expiratory volume) and FIV (forced inspiratory volume) have been suggested as indices of respiratory muscle function. Tables of normal values are available (Black & Hyatt 1969) and it has been suggested that malnourished patients have reduced pulmonary function which returns to normal with nutritional support (Grant 1980). However, normal pulmonary compliance and air-way resistance are implicit in these measurements which is frequently not the case in sick people.

Hand dynomometry is another measure of muscle function which has been suggested as a useful index of malnutrition (Klidjian *et al.* 1980), but once more sufficient data are not available.

Radioisotope methods

Total body nitrogen (Hill *et al.* 1978) or total body potassium (Boddy *et al.* 1972) are much more accurate methods of indicating lean body mass but both methods require expensive apparatus.

Laboratory measurements

Malnutrition affects all tissues. Most laboratory investigations reflect different influences and require considerable interpretation. The ideal of a single test of malnutrition is therefore impossible to achieve but plasma proteins have proved to be of greatest value.

Plasma proteins

Most plasma proteins, other than immuno-globulins are synthesized by the liver and have a varied response to malnutrition. Plasma albumin is commonly used as a marker of malnutrition and indeed low plasma levels often reflect malnutrition. Changes in plasma albumin levels however can be due to changes in circulating volume which accounts for most of the fall in plasma albumin commonly seen post-operatively. Furthermore, albumin's long half-life of 20 days makes it an insensitive barometer of malnutrition. Serum prealbumin, and retinol binding protein, with much shorter half-lives, are more sensitive indicators of malnutrition (Shetty *et al.* 1979; Young & Hill 1981).

Other laboratory tests

Anaemia is a common concomitant of malnutrition. Changes in a variety of measurements of immune status have been used to assess malnutrition and these are described in Chapter 10. Severe malnutrition is also associated with disordered liver function tests, but these tests are not diagnostic of malnutrition. Mineral and vitamin deficiencies may also require investigation.

ASSESSMENT OF NUTRITIONAL REQUIREMENTS

Having established from the history and examination that a patient needs nutritional support, it is necessary to decide what to give and how best to give it. Tables 1.3, 1.4 and 1.5 illustrate the framework for nutritional support though clearly the nitrogen and energy sources used depend on the route of administration.

Choice of route

It needs re-emphasizing that if a patient can be fed naturally then this is the method of choice, but if insufficient food is consumed then an alternative route is required. The failure to provide nutritious meals in an attractive manner is regrettably common in modern hospital practice. The development of a trayed meal service administered by auxiliary staff means that nurses relinquish their duty of caring for the patient's nutrition. Catering managers should be made more aware of the needs of patients and dietitians and nurses should be more concerned with the nutrition of general patients. For many undernourished or anorexic patients the prescription of small, frequent, nutritious meals is all that is required.

Liquid feed

Patients who find chewing and swallowing difficult or cannot take enough in the form of solid food can be managed successfully using liquidized food or proprietary liquid meals to supplement their diet.

Tube feeding

Patients who have a functioning gastrointestinal tract but lack the motivation or capacity to swallow food, can be fed by tube which provides an excellent means of instilling a complete liquid diet. There are now many preparations which can be used, and the development of a fine-bore flexible naso-gastric tube has considerably improved patient comfort and reduced reflux oesophagitis. A longer tube may be placed directly into the duodenum because duodenal and jejunal activity often recovers before the stomach. Fine-bore silastic tube feeding can also be used successfully at home (Allison 1986).

Tube gastrostomy and jejunostomy

Gastrostomy and jejunostomy tubes inserted at operation are an important, and much underused means of feeding patients particularly after major upper intestinal surgery, for example oesophagectomy and gastrectomy. Conventional balloon urinary catheters (12 or 14 FG) or fine-bore silastic tubes appear equally effective means of access.

INTRAVENOUS FEEDING

Parenteral nutrition is invasive, unphysiological and expensive. It is hardly surprising therefore that the literature abounds with the problems caused by this form of nutrition, but careful attention to detail and parenteral nutrition teams minimize these problems (Fischer 1980). This reminder serves to emphasize that parenteral nutrition should be reserved for those patients where there is no acceptable alternative and in those units where the necessary experience is available. Our preference is to use an infraclavicular subclavian vein access which allows a flexible prescription of hypertonic nutrients delivered from a 3 litre bag.

Others have suggested that satisfactory total parenteral nutrition can be achieved via peripheral veins (Grotte *et al.* 1980; Jeejeehboy & Close 1981). Intravenous isotonic amino acids administered through peripheral veins has also been shown to reduce the post-operative negative nitrogen balance compared to the conventional glucose electrolyte solutions. It has also been suggested that routine use of such amino acid solutions might delay or reduce the need for other nutritional support (Blackburn *et al.* 1980) but this is by no means proven and at present should not be used until further evidence is available and isotonic amino acid solutions become less expensive.

Parenteral feeding using a central line can also be successfully carried out at home for those patients who require long-term or permanent parenteral feeding. These patients can lead a virtually normal life, connecting themselves to the intravenous feeding system at night. Success requires a well-trained patient and expert hospital support.

Cyclical feeding

It has been suggested that periodic rather than continuous feeding more closely resembles the physiological pattern of normal meals (Page & Clibon 1980). Theoretically, this allows the normal hormonal changes associated with a meal and the rest between meals to take place. Further work is required to verify this hypothesis.

CHOICE OF NUTRIENTS

A few important principles govern the choice of nutrients.

1   The patient's calorie, protein, mineral and vitamin requirements are determined primarily by the patient's metabolic state and not by the method of delivery. For example, a severely burned patient who is hypermetabolic will need so much protein and calories whether they are given orally, by tube, intravenously or any combination of these methods.

2   The nutritional regime should be as simple, safe and economic as possible.

3   Intravenous nutrition should mimic, as far as practical, normal nutrition.

4   Adjustments are commonly necessary as a result of monitoring the patient's progress.

Nitrogen and calorie requirements

The nitrogen and calorie requirements are closely intertwined and they generally increase with increasing energy expenditure or metabolic rate. In turn, the metabolic rate increases with increasing severity of injury or illness (Elwyn 1980). An approximate estimate of nitrogen and calorie requirements for individual patients can be made from Table 1.3 based on patient's body weight with an appropriate increment for increasing metabolic rate. The advantage of this method is that the prescription is individually prescribed and theoretically suited to each patient.

We have found however that most patients can be fed satisfactorily using standard regimes with careful monitoring. Individual prescriptions are reserved for the few patients who are metabolically unstable, for example those with severe sepsis, multiple injuries or liver or renal failure.

A more precise estimate of metabolic rate is made by measuring oxygen consumption (Bartlett *et al.* 1977). This technique is valuable in patients who are clinically hypermetabolic and the method is now available in many intensive care units particularly on patients who are ventilated mechanically. An estimation of nitrogen need is made by measuring urinary urea excretion or urine total nitrogen excretion. Allowances have, of course, to be made for changes in blood urea and also nitrogen losses from wounds and the gastro-intestinal tract (p. 104). The calculated nitrogen need also gives a guide to the patient's energy requirements (Table 1.3).

Close monitoring should ensure that each patient's requirements are met. Both calorie and protein adjustments may be needed to maintain a positive nitrogen balance.

Table 1.3. (a) Percentage change in resting metabolic rate in different clinical conditions; (b) energy and nitrogen requirements in different clinical conditions (modified from Elwyn 1980).

(a)

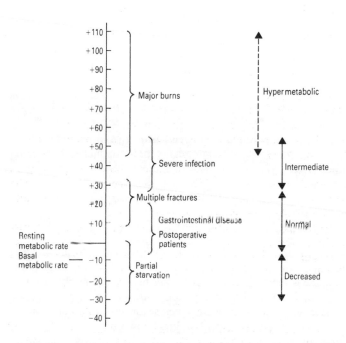

(b)

	Normal	Intermediate	Severely hypermetabolic
Energy per kg body wt	30 kcal (125 kJ)	35– 40 kcal (150–170 kJ)	40– 60 kcal (170–250 kJ)
Nitrogen per kg body wt	160 mg	200–300 mg	300–500 mg

Table 1.4. Recommended daily mineral intake for a 70 kg adult.

	Calcium mmol	Phosphorous mmol	Iron μmol	Magnesium mmol
Oral intake*	20	25	180–324	14
Absorption	20–30%		10–20%	About 40%
Intravenous intake†	7–14	14–70	21–70	7–28
AMA 1979 intravenous guidelines‡				
Signs of early deficiency	Low serum calcium NB interpretation depends on changes in albumin levels	Low serum and urine phosphorous concentrations	Microcytic anaemia. Low serum ferritin	Low serum and urine levels

*Food and Nutrition Board (1980) *Recommended Dietary Allowances* 9th edn. National Academy of Sciences, Washington D.C.

Calorie source

There are few difficulties supplying sufficient calories into the intestinal tract but the best calorie formulation for intravenous nutrition is controversial. There is now however general agreement that glucose is the best intravenous carbohydrate and there are no real advantages in using fructose or sorbitol. Fat alone is ineffective at inhibiting protein breakdown for gluconeogenesis, but administered with some glucose it appears as effective at maintaining a positive nitrogen balance as glucose alone. Current recommendations are to give glucose and fat in roughly equicaloric quantities (Elwyn 1980).

Insulin

Woolfson *et al.* (1979) have shown that the nitrogen balance in seriously ill hypermetabolic patients may be improved using glucose and exogenous insulin to maintain normo-glycaemia (p. 105).

Table 1.4. *continued*

Zinc μmol	Manganase μmol	Copper μmol	Chromium μmol	Floride μmol
230	45–90	30–45	1–4	78–208
About 60%	About 12%	30–80%	1–25%	
49–210	7–35	5–70	1	49
38–90	2.7–14.4	7.5–22.5	0.19–0.29	
Low serum and urinary zinc levels. Eczematous rash		Low serum copper and ceruloplasmin levels. Anaemia and leucopenia		

†Shenkin A and Wretlind A 1977 In Nutritional Support in the critically ill Ed. JJ Richards and J Kinney Churchill Edinburgh.

†American Medical Association. Department of Food and Nutrition (1979) *J Amer Med Ass*, **241**, 2051 2064

Nitrogen source

The best nitrogen source is whole animal and vegetable protein if the patient can eat normally. The same food may be blenderized for tube feeding or commercial preparations may be used instead.

Egg albumin has been used as the model to formulate intravenous amino acid mixtures. Glycine is often used as a major constituent, because it is cheap but it may not be a good source of amino nitrogen (Editorial, *Drugs and Therapeutic Bulletin*, 1980). However, at present there are no clear metabolic advantages for any one of the commercially available mixtures.

Essential fatty acids

The unsaturated fatty acid, linoleic acid, a constituent of all cell membranes and precursor of prostaglandins is an essential component of the diet. It is present in large amounts in corn, soya bean and sunflower oils and sufficient essential fatty acids will be given if about 2% of total calories are linoleic acid. 500 ml of 10% lipid

Table 1.4. *continued*

	Iodine μmol	Selenium μmol	Molybdenum μmol
Oral intake *	1.2	0.6–2.6	1.5–5.0
Absorption			
Intravenous intake†	1–7	0.4	0.2
AMA 1979 intravenous guidelines‡			
Sign of early deficiency	Biochemical tests for thyroid hormone		

See pages 12 and 13 for notes.

emulsion intravenously on alternate days, or 15 ml of sunflower oil orally or even massaged into the skin are sufficient.

Carnitine

Carnitine, which is normally synthesized in the liver (from lysine, methionine and glycine in the presence of ascorbate and pyridoxine) is necessary for the transport of fatty acids into mitochondria for oxidation. It is possible that exogenous carnitine may be of therapeutic value (Tao & Yoshimura 1980).

MINERALS AND VITAMINS

There are three main factors in assessing the needs for minerals and vitamins. Firstly, they may already be depleted for example due to a poor diet or malabsorption, secondly there may be increased requirements for tissue repair and thirdly there may be increased losses from the gut or wound drains etc.

Minerals

The major minerals, sodium, potassium and chloride are prescribed to maintain a normal fluid and electrolyte balance. Hypomagnesaemia and hypophosphataemia occur rapidly if these

Table 1.5. Recommended daily vitamin intakes for adults.

	Thiamin B_1 mg	Riboflavin B_2 mg	Niacin mg	Pyridoxine B_6 mg
Oral*	1.4	1.6	18	2.2
Intravenous†	3.0	3.6	40	4.0
Body store and time taken to deplete	No store	No store	Synthesised from tryptophan	
Signs of early deficiency	Red cell transketolase activity ↓ 15–20 days of deprivation	Stomatitis	Dermatitis	Non specific anaemia
Major dietary sources	Whole cereals Meat Potatoes Milk	Milk Meat Eggs Cheese	Meat Bread and Cereals Vegetables	Meat Fish Eggs Whole cereals

* Food and Nutrition Board (1980) *Recommended Dietary Allowances*, 9th revised edn National Academy of Sciences, Washington DC.
† American Medical Association. Department of Foods and Nutrition (1979) Multivitamin preparations for parenteral use. *Journal of Parenteral and Enteral Nutrition*, **3**, 258–262.

minerals are not added to parenteral nutrition solutions. Provision of trace elements is essential (Shenkin 1987). Although levels of intake have been recommended, further research is necessary to assess micronutrient status in the critically ill. Table 1.4 summarizes recommended daily intakes.

Vitamins

The body has negligible reserves of the water-soluble vitamins. These, and in particular folic acid, should therefore be given daily (p. 121). There are ample stores of the fat-soluble vitamins A, D, E in healthy people, but vitamin K may be depleted because of changes in gastro-intestinal flora. Vitamin K should therefore be given regularly to patients fed parenterally. Other fat-soluble vitamins should be given if parenteral feeding is to be prolonged.

Table 1.5 summarizes the recommended intakes, bearing in mind these are for healthy adults.

Table 1.5. *continued*

	Folate	Vitamin B_{12}	Pantothenic Acid	Biotin
	mg	μg	mg	μg
Oral*	0.4	3	4–7	100–300
Intravenous†	0.4	5	15	60
Body store and time taken to deplete	5–15 mg/kg in liver Main store liver 3–6 months	1–10 mg Main store liver lasts 3–6 years		Normally synthesized by gut bacteria
Signs of early deficiency	Red cell folate Megaloblastic anaemia	Serum level Megaloblastic anaemia	Not described	Dermatitis
Major dietary sources	Offal Green leafy Vegetables	Meat Fish Eggs Cheese	Widespread	Offal dairy products cereals

See page 15 for notes.

REFERENCES

Allison SP, (1986) How I feed patients enterally. *Proceedings of the Nutrition Society*, **45**, 163–169.

Bartlett RH, Allyn PA, Medley T & Wilmore IV (1977) Nutritional therapy based on positive calorie balance in burn patients *Arch Surg*, **112**, 974–980.

Beal VA (1967) The nutritional history in longitudinal research. *J Am Diet Ass*, **51**, 426–432.

Bistrian BR, Blackburn GL, Hallowell E & Heddle R (1974) Protein status of general surgical patients. *JAMA*, **230**, 858–860.

Black E (1981) Pitfalls in dietary assessment. *Recent Advances in Clinical Nutrition I*, p. 11, ed. Howard E & McLean Baird I. John Libbey, London.

Black LF and Hyatt RE (1969) Maximal respiratory pressures: Normal values and relationship to age and sex. *Am Rev Respir Dis*, **99**, 696–702.

Blackburn GL, Flatt SP & Hensle TW (1980) *Total Parenteral Nutrition*, p. 363, ed. Fischer JE. Little Brown & Co, Boston.

Boddy K, King PC, Hamek & Wyers E (1972) The relation of total body potassium to height, weight and age in normal adults. *J Clin Path*, **25**, 512.

Collins JP, McCarthy ID, Hill GL (1979) Assessment of protein nutrition in surgical patients—the value of anthropometrics. *Am J Clin Nutr*, **32**, 1527–1530.

Table 1.5. *continued*

Vitamin A μg	Ascorbic Acid C mg	Vitamin D μg	Vitamin K μg	Tocopherol E mg
1000	60	5	70–140	10
1000	100	5	0.03–1.5 per kg body wt	10
90–150 mg 90% in liver 75 days–1 yr	Exhaustion of body stores in about 29 days		No store Normally synthesised by gut bacteria	Wide distribution Stores said to be considerable
Poor dark adaptation Blood levels a poor guide Plasma levels maintained until severe deficiency	Leucocyte ascorbic acid concentration ↓	Blood levels reflect deficiency early Osteomalacia on bone biopsy	Decreased prothrombin time	
Fish liver oils Offal Eggs Dairy products	Citrus fruits Green vegetables Potatoes	Fatty fish Margarine Eggs Butter	Vegetables	

Cruse PJE and Foord R (1973) A five year prospective study of 23, 649 surgical wounds. *Arch Surg*, **107**, 206–211.

Dockel RC, Zwillich CW, Scoggin CH *et al* (1976) Clinical semistarvation depression of hypoxic ventilatory response. *New Eng J Med*, **295**, 358–361.

Durnin JV & Rahaman MM (1967) The assessment of the amount of fat in the human body from measurements of skinfold thickness. *Brit J Nutr*, **21**, 681–689.

Editorial (1980) Adult parenteral nutrition: which preparations? *Drug and Therapeutics Bulletin*, **18**(22), 85–88.

Elwyn DH (1980) Nutritional requirements of adult surgical patients. *Critical Care Medicine*, **8**, 9–20.

Fischer JE (1980) *Total Parenteral Nutrition*, p. 127, ed. Fischer JE. Little Brown & Co, Boston.

Forse RA & Shizgal HM (1980) The assessment of malnutrition. *Surgery*, **88**, 17–24.

Frisancho AR (1974) Triceps skinfold and upper arm muscle size norms for assessment of nutritional status. *Am J Clin Nutr*, **27**, 1052–58.

Grant J (1980) In *Handbook of Total Parenteral Nutrition*, p. 19. W.B. Saunders Company.

Grotte G, Jacobsen S & Wretlind A (1980) In *Total Parenteral Nutrition*, p. 335, ed. Fischer JE, Little Brown & Co, Boston.

Gurney JM & Jelliffe PB (1973) Arm anthropometry in nutritional assessment

—monogram for rapid calculation of muscle circumference and cross sectional muscle and fat areas. *Am J Clin Nutr*, **26**, 912–915.

Hill GL, Blackett RL, Pickford L, Burkinshaw L, Young GA, Warren JV, Schorah CJ & Morgan DB (1977) Malnutrition in surgical patients. *Lancet*, **i**, 689–692.

Hill GL, McCarthy ID, Collins JP & Smith AH (1978) A new method for the rapid measurement of body composition in critically ill surgical patients. *Brit J Surg*, **65**, 732–735.

Irvin TT & Hunt TK (1974) The effect of malnutrition on colonic healing *Ann Surg*, **180**, 765–772.

Jeejeebhoy KN & Close M (1981) Total parenteral nutrition by peripheral venous infusion. In 2nd European Congress on Parenteral and Enteral Nutrition, September 1980, ed. Wright PD. *Acta Chir Scand*, Suppl **507**, 419–420.

Jelliffe DB (1966) The assessment of nutritional status in the community. *WHO Geneva Monograph* **53**.

Klidjian AM, Koster KJ, Kammesling RM, Cooper A & Karran SJ (1980) Relation of anthropometric and dynamometric variables to serious post-operative complications. *Brit Med J*, **281**, 899–901.

Michel L, Serrano A & Malt RA (1981) Nutritional support in hospitalised patients. *New Eng J Med*, **304**, 1147–1152.

Nightingale F (1859, reprinted 1970) *Notes on Nursing*, p. 36. Gerald Duckworth, London.

Page CP & Clibon U (1980) Man the meal-eater and his interaction with parenteral nutrition. *JAMA*, **244**, 1950–1953.

Shenkin A (1987) Essential trace elements during intravenous nutrition. *Intens Therap Clin Monitor*, **8**, 38–47.

Shetty PS, Watrasiewicz KE, Jung RT & James WPT (1979) Rapid-turnover transport proteins: an index of subclinical protein-energy malnutrition *Lancet*, **ii**, 230–232.

Tao RC & Yoshimura NN (1980) Carnitine metabolism and its application in parenteral nutrition. *J Parenteral Enteral Nutr*, **4**, 469–486.

Todd EA, Hunt P, Crowe PJ, Royle GT, (1984). What do patients eat in hospital? *Human Nutr Appl Nutr*, **38A**, 294–297.

Woolfson AMJ, Heatley RV & Allison SP (1979) Insulin to inhibit protein catabolism after injury. *New Eng J Med*, **300**, 14–17.

Young GA & Hill GL (1981) Evaluation of protein-energy malnutrition in surgical patients from plasma valine and other amino acids, proteins and anthropometric measurements. *Am J Clin Nutr*, **34**, 166–172.

Chapter 2 · Basic Nutritional Background

The dietary components for man may be considered as energy, protein, vitamins, minerals and water.

ENERGY

Carbohydrate and fat are the major dietary sources of useful energy for the body but there is also a contribution from protein. The energy value is assessed in kilocalories (commonly referred to as 'calories') or, in S.I. units, kilojoules (1 kcal = 4.184 kJ).

Carbohydrate

Carbohydrates, normally taken as starches and sugars, are digested to monosaccharides, mainly glucose, prior to absorption. It is on various polymers of glucose that proprietary oral preparations are mainly based.

Alternative carbohydrate sources to glucose have been considered for intravenous feeding but have subsequently come into disfavour (p. 114). Glucose is the best carbohydrate for intravenous use, but unfortunately glucose solutions of high calorific value are hypertonic, and this causes venous damage. They must be infused only into a central vein and some patients may require insulin in addition.

Many patients can be fed intravenously with glucose as the main source of energy. Given at very high doses however, glucose may become less effective as an energy source. Some evidence for this is on p. 165.

Fat

Triglyceride is the form in which fats chiefly occur in food. The intestinal wall resynthesizes the fatty acids derived from fat digestion into triglyceride-protein—'chylomicra'—which enter the blood stream via the lymphatics.

Of the different intravenous triglyceride preparations tested, a stable triglyceride emulsion obtained from the soya bean has proved to be successful. Most research and clinical experience has been obtained with the product Intralipid. The Intralipid triglyceride has several properties that resemble natural chylomicra. Tissue uptake studies in normal subjects have indicated that muscle and adipose tissues are the main clearing sites of infused lipid with less clearance by the liver (Rössner 1974).

Very few side reactions have been reported from extensive experience of Intralipid in a wide range of diseases including trauma, burns, renal insufficiency and cachexia. There remains some controversy concerning the clinical complications of lipid and these are reviewed on p. 116. Lipid has the advantage over concentrated solutions of glucose as it is isotonic and can be infused via a peripheral vein.

Essential fatty acids

The fatty acid, linoleic acid, must be included in the diet and from this other unsaturated fatty acids can be synthesized which are essential for cell membrane integrity; they are also precursors of prostaglandins.

PROTEIN

An important aim of nutrition is to prevent breakdown of the body's proteins. There is no inert protein store: the bulk of skeletal muscle is the main protein reserve during starvation. However, if nutrition is deficient, not only is the patient weakened by the loss of skeletal muscle, but also tissue repair and immune mechanisms are significantly inhibited as these processes require active cell turnover and therefore new protein formation.

Protein is composed of amino acids and these can be considered in two groups: essential, i.e. those which cannot be synthesized by the body; and the non-essential amino acids. The essential amino acids are leucine, isoleucine, valine, methionine, threonine, lysine, histidine, phenylalanine, tryptophan and arginine. A comparison of different food proteins has shown that the efficiency of utilization, the 'biological value,' depends on the presence of sufficient amino acids: all of the essential amino acids plus enough of the other amino acids to meet nitrogen requirements.

Protein requirements can be considered in terms of the nitrogen content; protein loss from the body can be evaluated in the same way. As an approximation, 1 g of nitrogen is equivalent to 6.25 g of protein which since muscle is mainly water, is equivalent to about 32 g of muscle tissue.

The normal adult is in nitrogen balance; that is, the nitrogen retained from the food matches the nitrogen lost from the body: any extra nitrogen that is superfluous to body needs is excreted. The growing child, or the starving adult being refed, show a positive nitrogen balance. The under-fed patient must use his own skeletal muscle as a source of amino acids and enters a state of negative nitrogen balance unless the amino acids can be obtained by feeding.

There is a continuous turnover of body proteins with daily breakdown of skeletal muscle, to be replenished by new protein synthesis. There is a net loss of protein each day from the body which requires dietary replacement. The minimum daily needs for a healthy 70 kg man are approximately 42 g of protein (about 7 g of nitrogen). Nitrogen from protein that is metabolically broken down is excreted mainly in the form of urea and measurement of urine urea excretion is used as an index of body nitrogen loss.

Protein sparing

Consider the consequence of the body being deprived of food (Fig. 2.1). The carbohydrate store, liver glycogen is considerably depleted within 24 hours; the lipid stores from adipose tissue can however last for several weeks, therefore the body must become

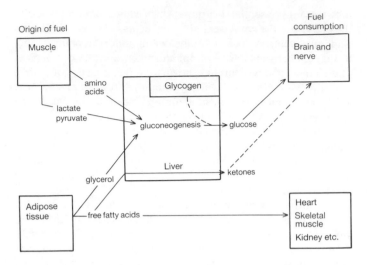

Fig. 2.1. The consequences of the body being deprived of food (modified from Cahill 1970).

mainly dependent on lipid for its energy needs. The blood glucose level is nevertheless maintained and the body must synthesize glucose during starvation (gluconeogenesis), as some tissues, especially the brain, depend on this glucose supply.

The source of substrate for gluconeogenesis is to a large extent amino acid derived from muscle. Initially, about 90 g of glucose are produced each day from amino acids and this reduces to about 16 g per day after about 5 weeks of starvation. This is because the brain and some of the other glucose-dependent tissues can adapt to use ketones as part of their energy supply.

The products of lipid mobilization are fatty acids, ketones (synthesized in the liver from partly oxidized fatty-acids) and glycerol. Fatty acids *cannot* be used for gluconeogenesis; glycerol provides substrate for about 19 g/day of new glucose synthesis (Newsholme 1976).

These factors explain why there is an accelerated net protein breakdown in starvation and also why giving small amounts of glucose but not lipid will result in reducing the need for this increased protein loss. Hence lipid alone *cannot* be used as the energy source; some carbohydrate or protein must be given in the diet to prevent the gluconeogenic protein breakdown.

It is suggested that about 500 kcal per day should be provided by carbohydrate and the rest of the calories can be given as either carbohydrate or lipid. These additional calories do have a further protein sparing effect, as demonstrated in healthy young adults where about 1400 kcal, approximately half the energy expenditure, was required for effective protein sparing when given with a basic protein intake (Elwyn 1980).

The findings described above relate to normal human subjects. The study of Jeejeebhoy (1976) showed that long-term intravenous feeding, providing total calories as 17% carbohydrate and 83% Intralipid, along with adequate amounts of amino acids, can successfully be given to patients with a variety of clinical conditions that require such nutritional support. Other clinical studies using different ratios of carbohydrate and lipid have confirmed these findings; use of a 1:1 ratio of carbohydrate and lipid is often recommended for intravenous feeding.

It is possible, particularly in the more stable obese patient, to give a hypocaloric regime in order to make use of the body's own fat stores. For the above reasons, a basic amount of carbohydrate should be supplied, and if necessary the nitrogen balance should be checked to ensure that effective protein sparing is maintained.

Choice of protein

Oral protein is digested to small peptides and amino acids prior to absorption. The intravenous nitrogen source must bypass the gut and is therefore given as amino acids. It has been shown that intravenous amino acids are utilized as efficiently as oral protein (Jeejeebhoy 1981).

Intravenous amino acid solutions were originally derived from protein hydrolysates but there are now commercially available mixtures of synthetic amino acids: the mixtures vary according to source but tend to approximate the amino acid composition of a protein of high biological value. Using the measure of nitrogen balance, the solutions from different commercial sources do not vary significantly in their clinical usefulness; increasing knowledge from the more complex measurements of amino acid utilization may help further define the amino acid concentrations optimal for intravenous use in ill patients.

There is, however, evidence that supplementation of branched chain amino acids can be beneficial in certain clinical cortexts. They are metabolized independently of the liver and furthermore may have a regulatory role in the promotion of protein synthesis and hence a possible usefulness in catabolic states. There is a disproportionate increase in circulating phenylalanine and tryptophan in the presence of liver cell failure. This leads to an imbalanced synthesis of neurotransmitter substances derived from these amino acids—a possible cause of hepatic encephalopathy. Providing branched chain amino acids can reduce the brain concentrations of phenylalanine and tryptophan by competition at the neutral amino acid carrier system of the blood-brain barrier. Some success has been reported in the reversal of encephalopathy consequent to the infusion of branched-chain enriched amino acid solutions (Sax *et al.* 1986).

VITAMINS AND MINERALS

Apart from the comparatively large requirements of the major minerals (sodium, potassium, chloride, calcium, magnesium and phosphate) the vitamins and minerals are required in trace amounts, but are nevertheless essential nutrients. Their involvement in metabolism is profound, for example by contributing cofactors to numerous enzymes. The recommended requirements in normal health are now relatively well defined but continue to be revised. For ease of presentation the information has been tabulated (pp. 12–17).

WATER

Water is of course an essential dietary component. Feeding actually increases the water requirement because more urine is produced to excrete the additional waste products.

THE NUTRITIONAL REQUIREMENTS OF ILLNESS

Tissue repair imposes demands on nutritional supply, and an increased activity of body defence mechanisms may also increase the nutritional needs. Despite this, ill-health is often associated with a decreased desire for food and decreased nutritional intake.

Various changes in the metabolism of carbohydrate, fat and protein can be observed in illness. Proportional to the severity of illness, there is an increase in the body's energy requirement and also an increase in the urinary nitrogen loss (Cuthbertson 1980). The scale of these changes is shown on p. 11. This response to illness has been termed a 'stress' response and the state of increased energy and protein needs, a 'hypermetabolic' state.

Hormonal changes appear to be important determinants of the stress response. Simply stated, insulin stimulates glucose uptake and metabolism, and glycogen, fat and protein synthesis. During starvation, insulin levels are low, and other hormones are effective in mobilizing body 'stores', that is they promote glycogen, fat and protein breakdown and stimulate gluconeogenesis and ketogenesis. In the stress response there is an increased secretion of this latter group of so-called 'catabolic' hormones, especially important being glucocorticoids, catecholamines and glucagon. The actions of insulin seem to be opposed by the catabolic hormones, an effect sometimes described as 'insulin resistance'.

Another fundamental event may be the production of the mediator interleukin-one a polypeptide produced by phagocytic cells including blood marocytes. An increasing number of direct effects, collectively termed the acute phase response, are now ascribed to this molecule including fever and the induction of muscle protein breakdown (Dinarello 1984).

In simple starvation, the metabolic breakdown of body fat is reversed by the feeding of glucose. In the hypermetabolic patient, it is found that fat breakdown continues despite giving glucose, and that gluconeogenesis and glucose oxidation also occur at increased rates. Hence the increased gluconeogenesis can increase the amount of carbohydrate that is required to obviate protein breakdown (see section on 'protein sparing').

To account for the increased nitrogen loss observed in stressed patients, there is both a depression of new protein synthesis and also an increase in the rate of protein breakdown (James 1981). Isotope measurements and studies of 3-methylhistidine excretion have contributed to these conclusions. 3-methylhistidine is present almost exclusively in skeletal muscle: furthermore, when muscle protein is broken down, it is not used further but is excreted in the urine, i.e. it can be used as a measure of the breakdown component of muscle protein turnover, and to help assess separately the effects of changes in protein breakdown or synthesis.

Three approaches to modifying protein synthesis or breakdown have received recent attention. Firstly, the addition of insulin may improve the effectiveness of nutrition in counteracting a negative nitrogen balance in the hypermetabolic patient. Secondly, the branched chain amino acids, particularly leucine may have a special ability to promote protein synthesis. Thirdly, there is a possible regulatory role of ketones in diminishing protein breakdown (Jeejeebhoy 1981).

Continuing research should further improve knowledge of the optimal amounts of carbohydrate, fat, protein, vitamins and minerals that are needed for the individual ill patient.

REFERENCES

Cahill GF (1970) Starvation in man. *New Engl J Med*, **282**, 668–675.

Cuthbertson DP (1980) Alterations in metabolism following injury. *Injury*, **11**, 175–189 and 286–303.

Dinarello CA (1984) Interleukin-one and the pathogenesis of the acute-phase response. *New Engl J Med*, **311**, 1413–1418.

Elwyn DH (1980) Nutritional requirements of adult surgical patients. *Crit Care Med*, **8**, 9–20.

James WPT (1981) Protein and energy metabolism after trauma. *Acta Chirurg Scand*, Suppl **507**, 1.

Jeejeebhoy KN, Anderson GH, Nakhooda AF, Greenberg GR, Sanderson I & Marliss EB (1976) Metabolic studies in total parenteral nutrition with lipid in man. *J Clin Invest*, **57**, 125–136.

Jeejeebhoy KN (1981) Protein nutrition in clinical practice. *Brit Med Bull,* **37**, 11–17.

Newsholme EA (1976) Carbohydrate metabolism *in vivo. Clin Endocrinol Metabol*, **5**, 543–578.

Rössner S (1974) Studies on an intravenous fat tolerance test. *Acta Med Scand*. Suppl **564**, 1–24.

Sax HC, Talamini MA, Fischer JE (1986) Clinical use of branched-chain amino acids in liver disease, sepsis, trauma and burns. *Arch Surg*, **121**, 358–366.

Chapter 3 · Pharmaceutical Aspects of Parenteral Nutrition

This chapter considers how to provide the prescribed intravenous nutrition; regimes for oral nutrition are in Chapter 6. The following aims are paramount in the preparation of TPN (total parenteral nutrition) infusions:

1 The maximum chemical and physical compatibility of all constituents during the whole of the useful storage life of the TPN solution

2 The maximum guarantee of sterility of the solution and delivery system

3 The minimal cost of producing the prescribed regime.

BASIC INGREDIENTS

The metabolic considerations in the choice of ingredients are discussed in Chapters 2 and 9.

Nitrogen sources

The tables on pp. 227–9 show the range and content of amino acid infusion solutions currently available in the UK. The choice should be made on the grounds of cost and pharmaceutical convenience. The following factors influence pharmaceutical convenience:

1 Usefully high amounts of electrolytes, e.g. sodium, potassium, and phosphate in the solution, minimizing or eliminating the need for aseptic addition of these electrolytes

2 The availability of an electrolyte-free version of the solution to give flexibility in addition of electrolytes, and

3 A wide choice of nitrogen content in association with the above permutations of electrolyte content.

Energy sources

Carbohydrate

Glucose (dextrose) provides 3.76 kcal/g and solutions containing 5, 10, 15, 30, 40, 50% and 70% are available as i.v. infusion solutions from commercial sources, in some cases with potassium chloride incorporated (see also p. 231).

Fat

Intravenous fat emulsion is a 10% or 20% aqueous emulsion of soya bean oil, providing 9 kcal/g fat. It is isotonic, but its compatibility with many potential TPN ingredients remains doubtful (Allwood 1984).

Medium chain triglycerides (MCT) have been used enterally for sometime, an intravenous fat emulsion containing MCT is now available, as a 10% or 20% aqueous emulsion of equal parts MCT oil and soya bean oil (see p. 226).

Electrolyte sources

The table on p. 230 shows a selection of convenient injection solutions of electrolytes which may be needed as supplements to the TPN solution to match a particular patient's needs. Most of them are commercially available, but others need to be prepared by a hospital pharmacy department.

Vitamin sources

The intravenous multivitamin preparations listed on pp. 232–3, are pharmaceutically convenient.

Water-soluble vitamins

The use of 'Parentrovite' has been criticized as it omits some vitamins and contains others in high quantities. There is, however, no evidence of overdose risk and greater quantities of vitamins than those normally recommended for healthy people may be necessary for ill patients. Supplementation with folate is essential (see p. 121). As pantothenic acid and biotin are also omitted by this regime, they should, where possible, be given orally. 'Solivito' can be used to maintain a complete i.v. regime as it supplies all water-soluble vitamins, but the quantity of each vitamin may be inadequate for the additional demands of illness. Water-soluble vitamins are normally suitable for incorporation into TPN solutions and folic acid (Sodium folate, Boots Ltd.) may be incorporated in this way, although significant losses of this vitamin may occur due to erratic absorption onto the wall of the plastic container (Lee *et al.* 1981) or due to precipitation (Allwood 1984).

Fat-soluble vitamins

These are vitamins A, D, E and K. Normally, the body has stores of Vitamin A and Vitamin D but during long-term feeding or when there is evidence of malabsorption these vitamins should be supplemented. A suitable regime would include:

1   Vitamin K, given i.m. weekly (10 mg phytomenadione B.P.), guided by the prothrombin time

2   Vitamin E, given i.v. (as 500ml 10% fat emulsion on alternate days), or as 'Multibionta'

3   Vitamin A, (especially in malabsorption or long-term feeding), given as 'Multibionta' i.v. when 'Vitlipid' is not being given

4   Vitamin D, (especially in cases of malabsorption or long-term feeding), can be given as 'Vitlipid' daily added to the fat emulsion. This will provide only maintenance amounts and will be inadequate where the patient is already frankly Vitamin D deficient; this may be aggravated by failure of activation in liver or kidney disease.

The multivitamin solutions Solvito N and Vitlipid N Adult (p. 232) have recently been marketed by KabiVitrum, they are based on the American Medical Association's intravenous recommendations (Shenkin 1986).

Essential fatty acids

These are supplied by the fat emulsion. When the latter is not given, a substitute is to massage daily 15 ml of sunflower oil into the skin (Press *et al.* 1974).

Trace elements

Shenkin *et al.* (1987) describes the use of Additrace (see p. 234), a mixture of nine trace elements designed to meet the increased needs of hospital patients.

In pharmacy-prepared regimes, the following can be added: chromium, copper, fluoride, iodide, manganese, selenium, and zinc. Adding 'Addamel' to a compatible amino acid or dextrose solution is an alternative, although concentrations per vial are low. Specially prepared pharmaceutical solutions will need individual formulation and stability testing (Kartinos 1978).

COMPOUNDING OF TPN SOLUTIONS

Apparatus

Accommodation

The area used to compound TPN solutions must ensure:
1   Their sterility
2   The minimal particulate content of these solutions.

Figure 3.1 shows a suitable lay-out. The air-supply to the clean room should be filtered to Class 1 standards (Code of Good Manufacturing Practice 1983) and the laminar flow cabinet must comply with the specifications for full aseptic manufacture and be large enough to accommodate all filling and compounding operations.

Sterile equipment

Apart from injection solutions, all sterile equipment is either disposable or re-autoclavable and drawn from the hospital Central Sterile Supply Department (CSSD).

Sterile clothing

Ideally, head caps, one-piece suits and face masks should be of low, lint-shedding nylon material (Code of Good Manufacturing Practice 1983) which is re-autoclavable (Burton *et al.* 1981). A fresh sterile outfit is used for each compounding session. In an emergency, theatre-quality sterile gowns, caps and face masks are acceptable. Plastic disposable overshoes must be worn in the clean area and on the clean side of the overshoe barrier of the ante-room. Gloves are disposable sterile plastic or rubber. As the hospital CSSD can usually prepare or provide this clothing, the pharmacy has to store only a small supply.

Special non-sterile equipment

Any special equipment of this type, e.g. drip stands, vacuum-bag filling machine must be thoroughly cleaned and disinfected with alcohol before being placed in the clean room. The *absolute minimum of apparatus* should be stored in this room.

TECHNIQUES OF PREPARATION OF TPN BAGS

Assembly of equipment

All apparatus and clothing needed for a given operation (checked against a master list) is assembled on a tray or trolley on the dirty side of the barrier (see Fig. 3.1). The apparatus is taken across the barrier onto the clean trolley in the ante-room, and in so doing it is either sprayed with 70% industrial methylated spirit (IMS) or the unsterile overwrap is discarded. The loaded clean trolley may be wheeled into the clean room. The operator must wash and disinfect his hands and arms and dress in sterile clothing in the ante-room.

The working surface of the laminar flow cabinet is thoroughly sprayed with 70% IMS and allowed to dry. Do not rely on the sterilizing action of an ultraviolet lamp fitted inside the cabinet. All equipment actually placed in the cabinet must be sprayed again with 70% IMS or placed directly in position from its sterile overwrap.

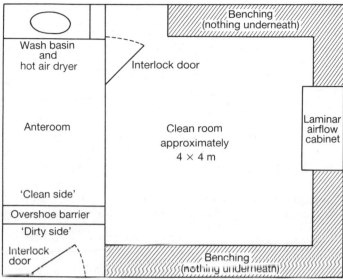

Fig. 3.1. Diagram of the TPN-compounding room.

Pharmaceutical Aspects

Compounding techniques

The process is in essence the aseptic transfer of sterile solutions from bottle, bags, or ampoules into a sterile large volume receiver with due consideration for the chemical and physical stability of the resulting mixture.

The receiver is usually a sterile plastic TPN bag of up to three litres capacity, with up to six attached tubes through which the contents of bottles/bags of constituents will flow. Each tube has a built-in airway incorporating a hydrophobic bacteriological filter to allow aseptic venting of rigid containers. The filling of the receiver can be either:

1   Under gravity

2   Aided mechanically by a vacuum-filling device

3   By means of a large-capacity syringe plus non-return valves ('Multi-Ad', Braun: 'Benja-Mix', Travenol)

4   By means of a programmable pumping device ('Vacuum', Pfrimmer-Viggo; 'Auto-Mix', Travenol).

The plastic receiver TPN bag may be of PVC, EVA, or combinations. The EVA type of bag is preferable as it eliminates the danger of leaching of plasticizers out of the bag into the TPN mixture (Allwood 1984; Farwell 1980).

Extra ingredients from ampoules or vials are injected through a suitable filter into the TPN bag *via* the injection port.

Typical TPN fluids are complex mixtures, and therefore drugs, electrolytes or trace elements must be added with extreme caution. The following principles should be applied to minimize the risk of precipitating sparingly soluble additives during the compounding process:

1   Add each additive separately

2   Inject into the running solution as it enters a bag which is nearly full so as to produce instantly the maximum dilution

3   Do not add any unnecessary additive or drug to the TPN solution as any new addition will need evaluation for stability. This problem is exemplified by the precipitation of Ca^{++} ions by the addition of souble bicarbonate or phosphate salts to the TPN solution (Fig. 3.2). Precipitation is related to the molar concentrations of calcium, bicarbonate or phosphate ions and to the resulting pH and the length of storage of the complete solution. To obviate this potential problem, the following must be noted:

1   Add, as above, the phosphate or bicarbonate salt before the calcium salt

2   Keep the pH as low as possible (Giovanoni 1976; Nedich 1978; Farwell 1980; see Fig. 3.2).

Other problems of incompatibility are theoretically possible and each TPN recipe should be analysed with this in mind.

Storage of prepared solutions

Once completely prepared, the TPN solutions should be infused into the patient during the next 24 hours.

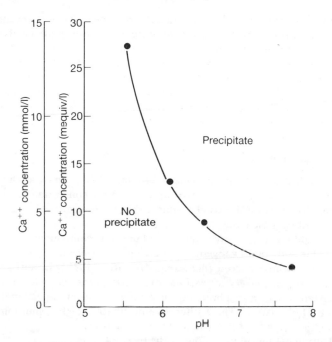

Fig. 3.2. Calcium ion concentration in a prepared TPN solution as a function of pH for calcium phosphate precipitation at 24 hours (after Nedich 1978).

The risks of microbial growth, especially of yeasts, are greatest once the TPN mixture has been completely prepared. A considerable variation has been reported however on the growth-supporting properties of various TPN recipes (Allwood 1984). Nevertheless, storage of these mixtures at 2–6°C almost eliminates growth of any contamination for many days (Duffet-Smith & Allwood 1979; Farwell 1980).

After compounding, the ingredients of the TPN mixture may degrade or be changed chemically or physically. Vitamins are particularly susceptible in this respect. Other TPN ingredients and physical conditions may influence these changes. The greater the complexity of the final TPN mixture, the more unpredictable the changes will be. Therefore, the increased convenience for the patient of having all ingredients in one TPN bag (e.g. incorporating lipid suspensions and drugs) must be balanced against the risks of unforeseen chemical and physical changes. Allwood (1984) has surveyed this subject and reference should be made to this very comprehensive review.

Presentation for ward use

The pharmacy should provide a 24-hour TPN regimen already fitted with the giving set, needing only simple connection to the patient by the ward staff. To achieve this, the pharmacy should at the last possible moment:

1 Add aseptically any vitamins and unstable compounds
2 Fit and connect together the giving sets needed. Giving sets with built-in 5 micron filters (e.g. 'Intrafix TPN' B Braun) are desirable to prevent a possible infusion of gross particles, e.g. slivers of rubber or plastic not detectable by visual inspection of the TPN mixture. These filters are unsuitable for fat emulsions which need a filter not smaller than 15 microns.
3 Seal off the additive port of the bag
4 Label the preparation (Fig. 3.3)
5 Cover the TPN bag with a light-proof cover, e.g. black or red plastic, to minimize the photolytic degradation of ingredients during infusion of the TPN mixture. Experimental giving sets and bags of coloured plastic are available (Avon; Miramed).

PARENTERAL NUTRITION SOLUTION

GLUCOSE	G	SODIUM	mmol
NITROGEN	G	POTASSIUM	mmol
VITAMINS	ml	CALCIUM	mmol
FOLIC ACID	mg	MAGNESIUM	mmol
		ZINC	mmol
TRACE ELEMENTS		CHLORIDE	mmol
		PHOSPHATE	mmol
TOTAL VOL.			

Fig. 3.3. An example of a TPN label.

6   Store the completed TPN bag at 4°C until delivery to the ward. There must be no warming of the refrigerated TPN preparation or fat emulsion to body temperature on the ward. The rate of infusion is fairly slow (*c*. 2.5 ml/min) and the fluid will warm up adequately while running through the giving sets.

Approximately 20–30 minutes of skilled pharmaceutical time is needed to prepare, ready for ward use, a TPN bag for infusion. Deep-freezing of TPN mixtures, including lipid components, may allow satisfactory storage for several weeks and thawing to a chilled temperature may be possible in a specially adapted microwave oven (Ausman *et al.* 1981).

Monitoring and quality-control

Microbiological

1   Blood Agar and Sabouraud Agar settle plates (previously appropriately incubated to eliminate false positive plates) should be exposed inside the laminar-flow cabinet and on nearby open benching during the whole compounding operation.

After further appropriate incubation, the following results are acceptable:

1   Plates exposed inside the cabinet = NIL colonies/60 min exposure
2   Plates exposed outside the cabinet = 5 colonies/60 min exposure.

The airflow in the cabinet must be measured with an anemometer at least every 3 months. The airflow rate must comply with the manufacturer's specification.

2   At randomly chosen times, the compounding process may be challenged by having the operatives transfer sterile nutrient broth into sterile containers using exactly the same apparatus and conditions used for the TPN compounding. The broth containers are then incubated as for sterility testing.

3   A keeping sample of 20–30 ml should be aseptically withdrawn from each complete bag. This can be placed in a sterile container or left in the syringe. Sterility can be done on a representative sample

and any residue reserved in a deep-freeze. The results of these tests can be used retrospectively to measure the quality of the compounding process, the actual TPN solution to which these tests refer having been used before the results become available. This situation parallels the preparation of short half-life radio-pharmaceuticals.

Chemical and physical

The keeping sample (see above) will also allow a retrospective analysis of the chemical and physical properties of the TPN solution, e.g. electrolyte and particle content. The effect of storage itself on these may be important (Farwell 1980).

In common with all i.v. solutions, an inspection just before use must include checks for leakage from containers, for particles, and for changes in appearance (Calvert & Goss 1984).

PHARMACEUTICALLY-PREPARED REGIME — AND ALTERNATIVES

The provision of the day's regime prepared in a single container by the hospital pharmacy or by a commerical compounding unit has the following advantages:

1 A regime to suit the patient, including the electrolyte needs
2 Significantly easier administration by the ward staff
3 Reduction of infection hazards
4 The various nutrients are mixed and given evenly throughout the 24 hours.

When the above series is not available, commercially available bottles of nutrient solutions must be used to which are added the vitamin and mineral supplements either in pharmacy or on the ward. A discussion of administering bottle regime is on p. 62.

The following are examples of possible regime (excluding the necessary vitamin and mineral additions). The regime for the particular patient should however be formulated according to the patient's needs using the information given in the text and in the Appendix.

A standard regime (2000 kcals; 14 g Nitrogen)*: TPN bag

Content		Example formulation	
Carbohydrate	250 g	Synthamin 14	1000 ml
Nitrogen	14 g	Nutracel 400	500 ml
Sodium	100 mmol	Dextrose 20%	500 ml
Potassium	100 mmol	Dextrose 10%	500 ml
Calcium	7.5 mmol	Sodium chloride 30%	5.5 ml
Magnesium	14 mmol	Potassium chloride	
Phosphate	30 mmol	15%	20 ml
Chloride	191 mmol	plus (separately)	
Zinc	0.04 mmol	Intralipid 20%	500 ml

A standard regime (2000 kcals; 14 g Nitrogen): equivalent in bottles

Content		Example formulation	
Carbohydrate	250 g	Synthamin 14	1000 ml
Nitrogen	14 g	Nutracel 400	500 ml
Sodium	75 mmol	Dextrose 20%	500 ml
Potassium	60 mmol	Dextrose 10%	500 ml
Calcium	7.5 mmol	Intralipid 20%	500 ml
Magnesium	14 mmol		
Phosphate	30 mmol		
Chloride	124 mmol		
Zinc	0.04 mmol		

A standard regime without fat (2000 kcals; 14 g Nitrogen)*: TPN bag

Content		Example formulation	
Carbohydrate	500 g	Synthamin 14	1000 ml
Nitrogen	14 g	Dextrose 50%	1000 ml
Calcium	11 mmol	Water for injection	500 ml
Sodium	100 mmol	Calcium chloride	
Potassium	100 mmol	13.4%	12.5 ml
Magnesium	19 mmol	Magnesium sulphate	
Phosphate	30 mmol	50%	7 ml
Chloride	160 mmol	Sodium chloride 30%	5.5 ml
		Potassium chloride	
		15%	20 ml

A standard regime without fat (1900 kcals; 12 g Nitrogen)*: equivalent in bottles

Content		Example formulation	
Carbohydrate	480 g	Aminoplex 12	1000 ml
Nitrogen	12 g	Glucoplex 1000	2000 ml
Sodium	140 mmol	Addamel	10 ml
Potassium	90 mmol		
Calcium	5 mmol		
Magnesium	8.5 mmol		
Phosphate	36 mmol		
Chloride	214 mmol		

A regime with low chloride (2000 kcal; 14 g Nitrogen)*: TPN bag

Content		Example formulation	
Carbohydrate	250 g	Synthamin 14	
Nitrogen	14 g	(electrolyte free)	1000 ml
Sodium	100 mmol	Nutracel 400	500 ml
Potassium	100 mmol	Dextrose 20%	500 ml
Calcium	7.5 mmol	Dextrose 10%	500 ml
Magnesium	14 mmol	Sodium acetate 34%	11 ml
Phosphate	15 mmol	Potassium phosphate	
Chloride	88 mmol	17.4%	15 ml
Acetate	103 mmol	Potassium acetate	
Zinc	0.04 mmol	49%	2 ml
		plus (separately)	
		Intralipid 20%	500 ml

*NB The above regime must be given with vitamin and mineral supplements.

REFERENCES

Allwood MC (1984) Compatibility and stability of TPN mixtures in big bags. *J Clin Hosp Pharm*, **9**, 181–98.

Ausman RK, Kerkof K, Holmes CJ, Cantwell BS, Kundsin RB, & Walter CW (1981) Frozen storage and microwave thawing of parenteral nutrition solutions in plastic containers. *Report, Dept of Surg, Med Coll* (Wisconsin. USA) & Travenol Labs, Derefield (Ill, USA).

Burton WR, Marshall IW, Metcalf B, & Taylor R (1981) Cleaning and disinfection of cleanroom garments. *Pharm J*, **226**, 30–1.

Calvert RT, & Goss I (1984) Paediatric Parenteral nutrition—pharmacy perspectives. *Clin Nutr News*, **2**, 3.

Department of Health and Social Security (1983) *Guide to Good Pharmaceutical Practice HMSO.*

Duffett-Smith J & Allwood MC (1979) Further studies on the growth of micro-organisms in total parenteral nutrition solutions. *J Clin Pharm*, **4**, 219-25.

Farwell J (1980) Pharmaceutical factors in long-term parenteral nutrition. *Proc Guild Hosp Pharmacists*, **8**, 3-40.

Giovanoni R (1976) *Total Parenteral Nutrition*, 27-54, ed. Fischer JE. Little Brown & Co, Boston.

Kartinos NJ (1978) Trace element formulations in intravenous feeding. *Advances in Parenteral Nutrition*, 233-40. ed. Johnston IDA. MTP Press, Lancaster.

Lee DR. Ware I & Winsley BE (1981) The survival of folic acid in total parenteral nutrition solutions. *J Intravenous Ther*, **1**, 13-16.

Nedich RL (1978) The compatibility of extemporaneously added drug additives with 'Travasol' (amino acid) injection. *Advances in Parenteral Nutrition*, 415-24, ed. Johnston IDA MTP Press, Lancaster.

Press M. Hartop J & Prottey (1974) Correction of essential fatty-acid deficiency in man by the cuutaneous application of sunflower-seed oil. *Lancet*, **i**, 597-9.

Shenkin A (1986) Vitamin and essential trace element recommendations during intravenous nutrition: theory and practice. Proceedings of the Nutrition Society **45**, 383-90.

Shenkin A, Fraser WD, McLelland AJD, Fell GS & Garden OJ (1987) Maintenance of vitamin and trace element status in intravenous nutrition using a complete nutritive mixture. *J Parenteral Enteral Nutr*, **ii**, 238-42.

Chapter 4 · Techniques of Administration of Parenteral Nutrition

INTRODUCTION

The ideal system for administration of total parenteral nutrition (TPN) would be longlasting, completely safe for the patient and economic of medical and nursing staff time. Such a system would have to overcome the related problems of sepsis and mechanical failure. The ideal is rarely approached in practice.

Often, the patient who needs TPN in a busy general ward is prescribed a complex, often inappropriate regimen based on a drug company advertisement. This regimen requires more than one feeding line, frequent bottle changes and constant vigilance. Hopefully an experienced member of staff is sought to insert the intravenous catheter. An anaesthetist is often asked because he is experienced in placing rigid central venous catheters for short-term venous pressure monitoring, but whoever is chosen will often have no subsequent direct interest in the functioning of this feeding catheter. The catheter itself is chosen at random from the ward store. A successful placement is effected, but the catheter later blocks, leaks, 'falls out' or, after a great deal of tampering, finally becomes infected. This experience leads doctors and nurses alike to regard TPN with apprehension. Thereafter TPN therapy is withheld from, or given only at a late stage to, patients who could benefit from it.

The establishment in 1978 of a TPN team in Oxford allowed a selection of equipment and a variety of techniques to be evaluated. The most successful of these were adopted as routine. Two surgical members of the team initially agreed to supervise the insertion of all central venous catheters to be used for TPN, whilst the specialist nurse accepted responsibility for management of the feeding line and catheter. A number of basic practical problems were identified and eliminated as the system evolved. This chapter describes the simple fluid administration system which was developed for TPN and outlines alternatives.

THE PROBLEMS

Catheter insertion

It is usual for articles on central venous catheterization to include long lists of recognized complications (Silk *et al*. 1978). Such lists rightly encourage caution in the use of central venous catheters for fluid administration and some authors have advocated the routine use of peripheral veins for parenteral nutrition. However, this places severe restrictions on the osmolality of infused fluids because the hypertonicity of TPN solutions produces thrombophlebitis in small veins whose blood flow is too low to dilute the solution rapidly. Even if solutions of relatively low osmolality are used, daily changes of the infusion site are necessary and debilitated patients rapidly run out of usable veins (Collin *et al*. 1975). Such a method can therefore only be used when the anticipated period of TPN is short and the metabolic requirements of the patient are low (Allardyce 1978).

To meet the requirements of most patients who need TPN, subclavian vein catheterization by the infraclavicular approach remains the method of choice. In this position the catheter occupies only a small proportion of the vein lumen, and fluids infused through it are diluted approximately 1000 times in their passage through the heart. Just like any other invasive procedure, this catheter placement should be carried out or supervised by an experienced operator. Complications are less common in the hands of those who have carried out 50 or more placements (Bernard & Stahl 1971). Restricting this procedure to a few members of the hospital staff will therefore pay dividends in keeping the complication rate low. Table 4.1 gives a list of complications together with hints for their avoidance. The commonest complication is pneumothorax which occurs in about 3% of cases in good hands. Many of the other complications, although less common, are potentially life-threatening.

Table 4.1. Some complications of catheter insertion and how to avoid them.

Infection	Maintain strict aseptic technique.
Pneumothorax, subclavian artery puncture and brachial plexus injury.	Keep needle horizontal and close to clavicle. Aim for suprasternal notch.
Intrapleural infusion.	Check intravenous siting of catheter tip by lowering fluid container.
Thoracic duct laceration.	Elect to use right side.
Air embolism	Maintain 20° –30° head down tilt during insertion.
Incorrect positioning of catheter	Do not infuse hypertonic solutions until check X-ray is examined.
Catheter embolism	Do not use a through-the-needle catheter.

Catheter failure

Intravenous catheters fail because of clotting of blood within the catheter, breakage of the catheter or its hub, or accidental displacement. Clotting of the catheter usually occurs because the giving line tap has been closed or because an empty fluid container has not been replaced. Arrangements which involve multiple giving lines or frequent bottle changes are prone to this problem.

The more rigid catheters, whilst excellent for central venous pressure measurement, are not ideal for TPN because they excite a tissue reaction and are thrombogenic. They tend to fatigue and crack after several days. Softer, non-reactive catheters made of silicone rubber are therefore preferable. A catheter hub which is fixed in the infraclavicular fossa is repeatedly stressed by movements of the shoulder, a factor which contributes to early catheter breakage. Shoulder movements, as well as stressing the catheter, also displace the dressings and expose the catheter to sepsis. When infection does supervene there is only a short distance between the skin entry site and the subclavian vein so that septicaemia can quickly follow. Partly for these reasons we always bury our catheters in a subcutaneous tunnel. Buried catheters are less inclined to 'fall out'; an additional reason for using this technique.

Control of infusion rate

When a large volume of fluid, either in a single container or in multiple bottles, is connected to a central venous catheter, there is a risk that accidental rapid overinfusion may occur. This possibility can be excluded by incorporating a flow-control device into the giving line or alternatively by employing an infusion pump. These devices also solve the problem of running the infusion to time.

Sepsis

Infection of the catheter or contamination of the giving line with consequent septicaemia is a disaster. Failure of aseptic technique (in catheter placement or line management) and frequent disconnections of the line (because of mechanical failure or the use of a multiple bottle system) both increase the risk of infection (Allen 1978). The addition of drugs to the fluid container or giving set by the ward staff carries a further risk of contamination (D'Arcy & Woodside 1973).

THE ANSWERS

Catheter insertion

Many makes and designs of catheter are now available for central vein catheterization. Most are suitable for placement in the subclavian vein using the infraclavicular approach described below. Current evidence suggests that catheters made of silicone-rubber will have lower sepsis and blockage rates and also that catheters which are buried in a subcutaneous tunnel for part of their length before entering the vein are more conveniently managed. The following account of catheter insertion therefore describes the technique currently used by the authors to insert a silicone-rubber catheter which is designed for tunnelling (Nutricath S, Vygon UK Ltd) but the principles involved in subclavian vein puncture are the same for all types of catheter.

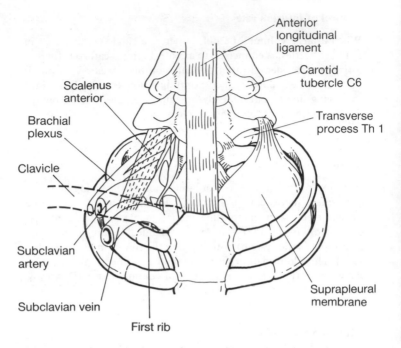

Fig. 4.1. The relationship of the right subclavian vein to the clavicle, first rib, scalenus anterior muscle and subclavian artery. The position of the suprapleural membrane is illustrated on the left side (after Last).

Catheter insertion by the infraclavicular approach

Full aseptic precautions must be taken during the insertion of central venous catheters. Non-sterile equipment is handled by an assistant. The procedure should ideally be performed in an operating theatre but can be carried out in a clean ward area provided that strict asepsis is maintained. The doctor should be aware of the anatomy of the thoracic inlet shown in Fig. 4.1 and it is important to explain the purpose and steps of the procedure to the patient before starting. Having 'a drip put into a vein just under the collar-bone' will not alarm the majority of patients and it is not usually necessary to give intravenous sedation.

A sterile trolley is prepared and the necessary equipment assembled (Table 4.2). A 500 ml bottle of saline is connected to a giving set with a luer lock and 'run-through' as for a normal intravenous infusion. The packet containing the sterile 45 cm extension set is opened at one corner only, to allow the female end of the extension set to be extruded and connected to the giving set. The rest of the extension set is left untouched within its packet, but is filled with saline from the giving set so that it is ready for connection to the catheter when this has been inserted.

The operator scrubs up, and is masked, gowned and gloved. If necessary the patient's chest and neck are shaved, any pillows are removed and he is then placed in a steep (20–30°), head down position with his head turned away from the side of catheter insertion. The shoulders should be drawn back slightly and occasionally, especially in the unconscious patient, a rolled up towel between the shoulder blades is helpful. The neck, right shoulder and anterior chest wall are painted with povidone-iodine solution (Fig. 4.2). Sterile drapes are applied, leaving exposed a square area which includes the suprasternal notch and right clavicle as far as

Table 4.2. Equipment for central venous catheterization

1 × 35 cm silicone feeding catheter plus spare (Vygon Nutricath S 2180.20)
2 × 10 ml syringes
1 × 21 G needle
1 × 23 G needle
10 ml 1% plain lignocaine
10 ml saline for injection
Sterile dressing pack containing:–
  gallipot
  2 pairs of forceps
  cotton wool balls
  gauze squares
1 × No 11 scalpel blade
1 × 3/0 nylon suture on a cutting needle
1 × sterile adhesive membrane
Pair of sterile suture scissors
Sterile drapes
Pair of sterile artery forceps
Povidone-iodine solution 10% w/v
Povidone-iodine dry powder spray

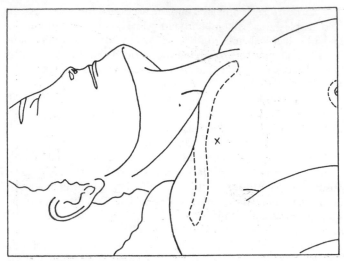

Fig. 4.2.

the delto-pectoral groove, and the chest wall for 15 cm below the clavicle (Fig. 4.3).

The point chosen for initial insertion of the catheter is 1 cm below the clavicle, just lateral to the clavicular head of pectoralis major (point X in Fig. 4.3). This is the medial limit of an easily palpable hollow below the clavicle; the delto-pectoral groove. The skin and subcutaneous tissues at this point are infiltrated with plain 1% lignocaine using a 23 G needle. The syringe and needle are then turned through 90° and the subcutaneous tissues are infiltrated with lignocaine for 8 cm in a line towards the umbilicus. This track will form the subcutaneous tunnel and at its caudal end (point Y in Fig. 4.3) the skin must be infiltrated so that sutures can be inserted later to hold the catheter hub in place. A 21 G needle, on a 10 ml syringe half-filled with saline, is advanced from point X towards the tip of the operator's left index finger which is placed gently in the patient's suprasternal notch (Fig. 4.4) The needle should pass almost horizontally, immediately behind and virtually

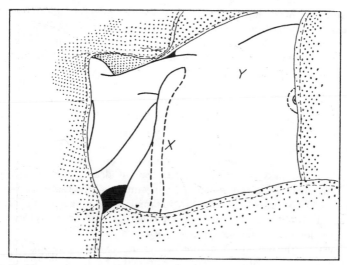

Fig. 4.3.

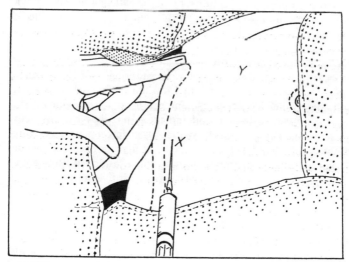

Fig. 4.4

parallel to the medial third of the clavicle, reaching the subclavian vein roughly midway between the skin entry point and the suprasternal notch. Occasionally, if the shoulder is prominent and cannot be drawn back, it may be necessary to use a more medial skin puncture site and to angle the needle slightly headwards. Gentle suction is applied intermittently to the syringe as the needle is advanced through the tissues. If strong or continuous suction is used, the lumen of the needle can become blocked with a plug of tissue. Free aspiration of blood into the syringe occurs when the vein has been entered and a mental note can then be made of the direction of the needle before it is removed. If the vein is not found on the first pass, the needle should be withdrawn completely, flushed with saline and inserted again, aiming a little more headwards. The subclavian artery, brachial plexus and lung apex all lie behind the scalenus anterior muscle (Fig. 4.1) and are therefore safe so long as the needle remains horizontal.

Seeking the vein with a fine needle in this way reduces the number of passes of the 14 G needle needed for catheter insertion and so minimizes complications, but if the patient is heavily-built it is sometimes impossible to reach the vein and a spinal needle, if available, can be used.

A 5 mm skin-crease incision is made at the skin entry point (X in Fig. 4.3). The cannula and needle assembly of the catheter placement kit is mounted securely on a 10 ml syringe containing saline and is advanced through the incision along the path previously followed by the 21 G needle. Again, gentle suction is applied to the syringe until a rush of blood indicates that the vein has been entered. A slight 'give' of the tissues often accompanies puncture of the vein. If arterial blood enters the syringe the needle should be withdrawn and the procedure temporarily abandoned. Pressure is then applied with a finger over the artery for five minutes and the head of the bed raised.

Once the needle tip is within the vein it should be advanced a further 3 mm or so, bringing the whole of the bevel into the lumen. The cannula is then eased forwards over the needle and into the vein after which the syringe and needle are withdrawn (Fig. 4.5). The patient can be instructed to perform the Valsalva manoeuvre

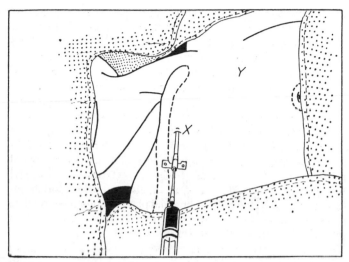

Fig. 4.6.

at this point to increase intrathoracic pressure and eliminate any risk of air embolism but not all patients find this easy, and hyperinflation can cause the lung apex to bulge into the root of the neck where it is in danger of being punctured during catheter insertion. For this reason patients being given intermittent positive pressure ventilation should have their ventilation momentarily suspended during passage of the needle. When the patient is placed 20–30° head-down there is always sufficient venous pressure to prevent air entry through the cannula, and the operator's left thumb has to be placed over the end of the cannula to prevent excessive blood loss rather than air entry.

The silicone-rubber catheter is passed through the cannula until it is 6 or 7 cm into the vein before its nylon stilette is removed (Fig. 4.6). Any difficulty in withdrawing it suggests that the line has passed up towards the neck. This can usually be prevented by tilting the head towards the shoulder on the side of catheter insertion. The catheter should be withdrawn a few centimetres and

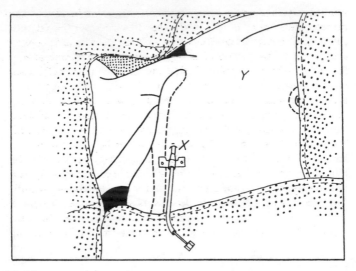

Fig. 4.6.

reinserted. The catheter is then advanced again until its tip is well
into the vena cava. This distance can be estimated by holding the
stilette against the patient. The catheter should pass easily. If it is
difficult to advance, then the catheter has usually become snagged
on the vein wall or the mouth of a tributary. A slight upward or
downward angulation of the cannula, or tilting the head again
often allows the catheter to pass more easily and the Valsalva
manoeuvre can sometimes help by distending the veins further. If
the catheter still will not pass, then the cannula should be withdrawn and a repeat venepuncture performed.

Five failed passes of a 14 G needle should be the maximum
allowed before abandoning the procedure, at least temporarily,
for fear of causing complications. No further attempt should be
made to cannulate the same or the contralateral subclavian vein
until a chest radiograph has been taken and examined to exclude a
pneumothorax.

When the catheter has been successfully introduced into the
vena cava the cannula is removed over the catheter and a pair of

small artery forceps temporarily applied to the catheter tip. The catheter must next be placed in the previously prepared subcutaneous tunnel. To do this the cannula and needle are reunited and passed percutaneously into the tunnel at point Y emerging at the infraclavicular incision beside the catheter (Fig. 4.7). Care must be taken not to lacerate the catheter with the needle as it is brought through the incision. The needle is once again withdrawn leaving the cannula in the tunnel. The artery forceps are removed from the catheter tip which is passed down inside the cannula until it appears at Y (Fig. 4.8). The cannula can then be removed finally, leaving only the catheter in the tunnel, and this is drawn out of the skin puncture site Y until the loop at X disappears (Fig. 4.9). The catheter should protrude 3 cm from Y for attachment of the hub. Any excess is cut off with sterile scissors so as to avoid leaving a redundant loop of catheter which can kink and occlude. This also removes the tip of the catheter which has been damaged by the

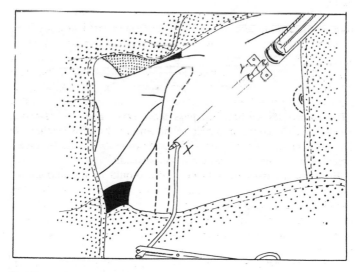

Fig. 4.7.

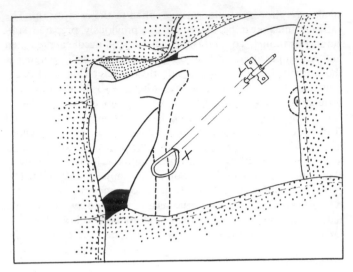

Fig. 4.8.

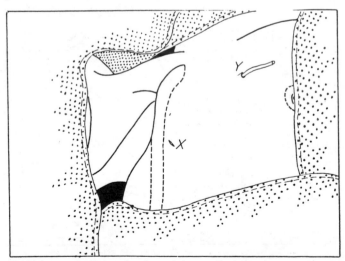

Fig. 4.9.

artery forceps. The hub is attached to the catheter as shown in Fig. 4.10.

The assistant peels open the packet containing the saline-charged sterile extension set allowing this to be taken by the operator who connects its male end to the catheter hub. The drip should now run freely, and the return of blood into the extension set when the saline bottle is lowered beneath bed level will confirm intravenous siting of the catheter tip. Saline is allowed to drip slowly until a check radiograph has been examined.

Two monofilament nylon sutures are used to fix the catheter hub to the skin. They should be tied loosely to avoid damaging the skin. A third nylon stitch or a steristrip closes the infraclavicular incision. Monofilament nylon sutures are particularly suitable because they are non-reactive and are resistant to infection. The skin puncture and suture sites are sprayed with povidone-iodine powder and small sterile gauze swabs are placed over the skin incision and catheter hub.

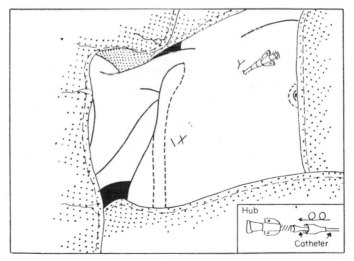

Fig. 4.10.

Finally, the patient's right arm should be abducted with the head still turned to the left and a suitable adhesive dressing is applied to seal the area, pinching it around the extension set tubing which can be looped up towards the shoulder under the dressing for extra security. When applied in this 'stressed' position adhesive dressings are less liable to subsequent displacement. The hub connection is now completely protected but the female end of the extension set remains outside the dressed area so that changes of the giving line can be performed without disturbing the catheter or its occlusive dressings (Fig. 4.11).

A good quality chest radiograph in expiration is taken as soon as possible after catheter insertion to confirm the catheter's position and to exclude a pneumothorax. This radiograph must be examined by the operator before any feeding solution is given. If the position of the catheter is in doubt, radio-opaque contrast medium can be injected down the catheter and a further radiograph taken. The catheter tip should lie in the superior vena cava or

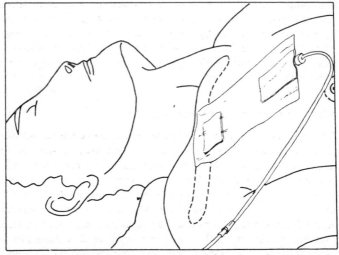

Fig. 4.11.

the upper portion of the right atrium. Provided that a silicone-rubber catheter is used, and that it follows the correct course, the precise position of the tip is not important. If a more rigid catheter is used then its tip must lie outside the attachments of the pericardium to avoid the risk of atrial perforation and cardiac tamponade (Greenall *et al.* 1975). If the catheter takes an aberrant course, passing for example up the internal jugular vein, then it may be possible to withdraw it to the subclavian vein but it is probably better replaced since venous thrombosis may follow infusion of TPN solution into too small a vein (Souter & Mitchell 1982).

Pneumothorax is the commonest complication of subclavian vein catheterization and although each one should be treated on its merits the majority are small and require neither chest drainage nor removal of the catheter. Repeat chest radiographs will be needed to ensure that the pneumothorax resolves. A small pneumothorax may not be evident on the first radiograph and shoulder-tip pain may be the only sign that anything is amiss. Patients who are given TPN in preparation for surgery should have a second chest radiograph in the 12 hours before operation to exclude the late appearance of a pneumothorax since this can be converted to a tension pneumothorax by intermittent positive-pressure ventilation (Mitchell & Steer 1980). Prophylactic chest drainage or other appropriate precautions should be taken during anaesthesia if the problem is anticipated.

Alternative methods of catheter insertion

The supraclavicular approach to the subclavian vein is sometimes preferred because it has been said to have a lower complication rate, however, it makes subcutaneous tunnelling more difficult.

If burns or the risk of infection from a tracheostomy make subclavian vein catheterization impossible or undesirable, or if the doctor is not experienced in the technique, a drum-loaded silicone-rubber feeding catheter (Intrasil, Travenol) can be passed centrally from the basilic (medial) vein in the antecubital fossa into the superior vena cava. Full aseptic precautions should be taken during insertion and a post-insertion chest radiograph is required to verify correct positioning of the catheter tip. This method does not carry the same risk of serious local complications as direct subclavian vein puncture, but threading the catheter all the way to the superior vena cava can be difficult and is often impossible. Care must be taken not to withdraw the catheter through the needle since this can cause shearing and embolism of the catheter itself. Antecubital lines have a high incidence of thrombophlebitis and sepsis and are difficult to dress securely. They are also more restricting for the patient, particularly since drum-loaded catheters are designed for insertion from the right arm.

A silicone-rubber catheter can be inserted in the cephalic vein under direct vision via a small skin incision. The vein is located in the mid upper arm using a Doppler probe. The catheter is passed up as far as the superior vena cava and the distal end tunnelled subcutaneously on the lateral side of the upper arm where it is secure and does not interfere with the patient's movements.

External and internal jugular vein catheters are generally less satisfactory for TPN administration than subclavian vein catheters because they are more difficult to dress adequately and restrict neck movements.

A variety of other approaches has been used with limited success. Catheterization of leg veins was found to be unsatisfactory because of the high sepsis rate. Even the inferior epigastric vein has been used for long-term home parenteral nutrition (Solassol and Joyeux 1976) but the buried subclavian vein catheter is by far the most popular for this purpose also. For home TPN however, a larger bore silicone-rubber catheter (Broviac or Hickman) is used and is usually inserted by an open surgical technique.

If a hubless catheter is not available but tunnelling is required, then a polyvinyl catheter can still be placed in a subcutaneous tunnel with the aid of a Seldinger guide wire which is usually available from the X-ray department. The floppy end of guide wire is positioned in the superior vena cava and the wire is then buried exactly as described for the hubless silicone-rubber catheter except that a 2–3 mm skin incision is made at the lower end of the tunnel (point Y in Fig. 4.3). When the cannula is removed after tunnelling, the catheter can be slipped onto the guide wire and pushed gently over it through the subcutaneous tunnel and into the vein. Once the catheter is in place the wire is removed and blood is aspirated from the catheter with a syringe to ensure intravenous placement and removal of air from the catheter. The catheter is then connected to a saline drip. This technique can also be used to replace a cracked catheter by passing a guide-wire through the old catheter before it is removed and sliding a new catheter over the wire into the vein. Unfortunately silicone-rubber catheters are too flexible to be pushed through the tissues in this way.

It is particularly important in patients with chronic or relapsing diseases such as Crohn's disease, to preserve superficial veins for vascular access. Care should be taken to ensure that venepuncture of any kind in such patients is carried out by a competent member of staff.

Catheter failure

The commonest line problem is blockage. This often happens when the patient is moved to the radiology department, operating theatre or elsewhere in the hospital where staff are unaware of the importance of keeping the line running. Patients leaving the ward should go with clear instructions about the line, either as a label attached to it or by giving clear instructions to accompanying staff.

Blocked lines may be cleared by placing the patient head down and under fully aseptic conditions (mask, gloves etc.) disconnecting the end of the extension set and flushing with saline in a 10 ml syringe. Pressure should be increased slowly on the plunger of the syringe until a sudden decrease in resistance indicates clearance of the line. If this does not work, a second attempt using a smaller syringe may be successful. Flushing with 'Hepsal' sometimes helps if the line is only partly blocked, causing the infusion to slow down. Streptokinase or urokinase may be used if these other methods fail (Hurtuboise *et al.* 1980). Lines which have been turned off for several hours may be impossible to unblock and need replacing. If a patient is to receive TPN for only part of the day the line can be kept patent by instilling with 5 ml 'Hepsal' before plugging it off.

Hubs or extension sets which crack should be replaced as soon as possible without disturbing the line, because of the risk of infection.

Occasionally the line slips out of the vein, either because it was inserted for only a short distance or because of traction on the line where it emerges from the tunnel. Suspicion is usually aroused by swelling around the shoulder as fluid accumulates in the soft tissues or by leakage from the tunnel into the dressings. If necessary, a chest radiograph can be used for confirmation. The line should be removed completely and, if necessary, replaced on the other side.

The most important point of line care is education of those most closely involved in the patient's care, including night staff. Ideally, if problems arise with which they cannot cope, there should be some nominated person readily available to whom they can turn for advice.

Flow control devices—accuracy versus economy

The infusion of large volumes of hypertonic solution calls for careful control of the rate of flow. Five types of flow control device are available and their cost increases with increasing accuracy.

Simple clamps

A simple but secure adjustable clamp applied to the giving line will give acceptable control in some circumstances. The appropriate drip rate is determined and set at the start of the infusion but must be checked regularly.

Since drop size varies with viscosity the drip rate required to give the same rate of infusion will vary from solution to solution.

Changes in the height of the fluid container relative to the patient, for example when the patient sits up or gets out of bed or as the fluid level in the container falls, result in changes in the drip rate. Though cheap, this method of flow control lacks safety and accuracy.

Variable resistance devices incorporated into the giving line

Devices of this type (e.g. Dial-a-flo, Abbott Laboratories) are also sensitive to viscosity changes and depend on a constant hydrostatic pressure to maintain constant flow. They are therefore subject to the same inaccuracies as a simple clamp but can be recalibrated for solutions of known viscosity.

Since the device forms an integral part of the giving line it cannot be accidentally removed.

An injection port on the distal portion of the device can be modified for the routine administration of lipid or for additional fluid replacement in patients with high fluid losses. These minor advantages probably fail to justify the expense of such devices for routine use, although they can be useful expedients in the short term.

Gravity-fed pressure-compensating devices (e.g. Isoflux, Geistlich)

These devices are sold as an integral part of a complete giving set and contain a flexible diaphragm which partially compensates for changes in hydrostatic and venous pressures giving some additional accuracy.

Electronic gravity-fed controllers (e.g. Accudot, Imed)

In this system a variable resistor, incorporated into the giving set, is adjusted automatically by an electronic controller. The controller monitors the drip rate using an optical drip counter attached to the drip chamber, and this feedback mechanism maintains a constant drip rate. Although a change in fluid viscosity will change the flow rate, changes in patient position or venous pressure do not. The system alarms for line occlusion or when the fluid container is empty. The cost of the special giving sets is comparable to that of conventional sets so that the extra expense lies in the purchase or hire of the electronic controller. The device is thus competitively priced for the degree of accuracy it offers. One advantage it holds over the volumetric pump is that the infusion continues at roughly the prescribed rate if the power unit fails.

Volumetric pumps (e.g. Imed 960)

These pumps provide highly accurate control of infusion by pumping measured volumes of fluid through a syringe mechanism. They are essential for the accurate infusion of small volumes, as in neonatal or paediatric work, but the power unit and special giving sets are expensive and some expertise is needed to set up the infusion initially.

Fluid containers

The potential advantages of the 'big bag' of mixed nutrients prepared by the pharmacy (see Chapter 3), are that the amino-acids and calorie source are delivered simultaneously and that, by spreading the dextrose load over 24 hours, rather than infusing high concentrations over shorter periods, the incidence of glycosuria is reduced (McGeehan *et al.* 1978). In addition, by minimizing the frequency of line disconnections and thereby the opportunity for contamination, the sepsis rate can be reduced (Allen 1978).

Until the benefits of cyclical administration of TPN, in which glucose is witheld for a period of 8 to 12 hours each day, are more clearly demonstrated, it seems likely that the advantages of a simple giving system are to be preferred, particularly for periods of TPN of less than 4 weeks (Benotti *et al.* 1976).

If a three litre container is not available, then some form of multiple bottle system will be necessary. However this is organized, it is important to minimize the number of connections and other potential sites of contamination if a high sepsis rate is to be avoided. In particular, 'piggy-backing' and the use of three and four-way taps is to be condemned (Freeman & Litton 1974).

Travenol manufacture two and three-lead (V and W) fluid administration sets whose leads are fused near the distal connector site. The bottles should be connected taking aseptic precautions and only the final connection needs to be made at the bedside. These administration sets have no injection ports or taps to encourage sabotage. Lipid emulsion can be infused via the lead which joins the system furthest downstream. Some expertise is required to limit the refluxing of one solution into another line, especially when lipids are in use. Alternatively, lipid emulsion can be given separately via a peripheral vein because it is almost isotonic and does not cause troublesome thrombophlebitis.

Sepsis

Redness of the skin overlying the tunnel may indicate infection tracking alongside the line. Swabs should be taken from the line exit site and either antibiotic treatment started (antistaphylococcal treatment is usually appropriate while awaiting the culture report), or the line removed depending on the patient's condition. Occasionally skin redness arises because of allergy to the dressing material and this should be suspected if it starts within 48 hours of inserting the line. A satisfactory alternative dressing can usually be found.

Patients developing septicaemia while on TPN should have blood cultures taken via the line and an alternative source of infection sought as quickly as possible by chest radiograph, urine culture etc. Antibiotic treatment should be started and if there appears to be no source of infection other than the line, it should be removed and the tip sent for culture.

The Oxford parenteral nutrition team does not use additional bacterial filters in its administration system. A pore size of 0.22 microns is required to filter out bacterial contaminants reliably. Such filters present a high resistance to fluid flow making it necessary to use an infusion pump. They are probably unnecessary if appropriate aseptic techniques are employed in the handling of fluids and equipment and may even lead to contamination since they represent a potential break in the giving line.

IN CONCLUSION

The dangers and pitfalls of TPN administration outlined in this chapter and discussed elsewhere in this book, underline the need for attention to detail in the safe administration of TPN therapy.

This chapter has described the equipment and techniques we find reliable and trouble-free. Although alternative methods have been included, it is our opinion that each departure from the preferred techniques will demand added vigilance on the part of the patient's medical and nursing attendants if the advantages of TPN are to outweigh the disadvantages.

Conversely, the introduction of a simple administration system can make TPN so apparently routine that its potential dangers are overlooked. The indications for TPN must be clear in each case before treatment is started (Chapter 1) and careful monitoring must be continued throughout (Chapter 7).

REFERENCES

Allardyce DB (1978) Clinical experience of total parenteral nutrition. *Advances in Parenteral Nutrition*, ed. Johnston IDA, 429–43. MTP Press Ltd, Lancaster.

Allen JR (1978) The incidence of nosocomial infection in patients receiving total parenteral nutrition in Johnston IDA (ed.) *Advances in Parenteral Nutrition*, 339–77. MTP Press Ltd, Lancaster.

Bernard RW & Stahl WM (1971) Subclavian vein cathetherisations: a prospective study. *Ann Surg*, **173**, 184–90.

Benotti PN, Bothe A, Miller JDB, Bistrian BR & Blackburn GL (1976) Cyclic hyperalimentation. *Compr Ther*, **2**, 27–36.

Collin J, Constable FL, Collin C, & Johnston IDA (1975) Infusion thrombophlebitis and infection with various cannulas. *Lancet*, **ii**(7926), 150–3.

D'Arcy PF & Woodside W (1973) Drug additives: A potential source of bacterial contamination of infusion fluids. *Lancet*, **ii**(7820), 96.

Freeman JB & Litton AA (1974) Preponderance of gram-positive infections during parenteral alimentation. *Surg Gynecol Obstet*, **139**, 905.

Greenall MJ, Blewitt RW & McMahon MJ (1975) Cardiac tamponade and central venous catheters. *Br Med J*, **2** (5971), 595–7.

Hoshal VL (1975) Total intravenous nutrition with peripherally inserted silicone elastomer central venous catheters. *Arch Surg*, **110**, 644–6.

Hurtuboise MR, Bottino JC, Lawson M and McCredie KB (1980) Restoring patency of occluded central venous catheters. *Arch Surg*, **115**, 212–13.

McGeehan D, Radcliffe AG, & Fielding LP (1978) Comparison of glucose homeo-stasis in total parenteral nutrition using small- and large-capacity containers. *Br J Surg*, **65**, 818-9.

Mitchell A, & Steer HWS (1980) Late appearance of pneumothorax after subclavian vein catheterisation: an anaesthetic hazard. *Br Med J*, **281**(6251), 1339.

Silk DBA, Lieberman DP & Sharrot P (1978) Parenteral nutrition. *Hospital Update*, **4**(10), 611-21.

Solassol C & Joyeux H (1976) Ambulatory parenteral nutrition in JE Fischer (ed.) *Total Parenteral Nutrition*, 285-301, Boston: Little Brown & Co.

Souter RG and Mitchell A (1982) Spreading cortical venous thrombosis due to infusion of hyperosmolar solution into the internal jugular vein. *Br Med J*, **285**(6346), 935-6.

The illustrations in this chapter were drawn by Mr Tony Wiseman of Vygon (UK) Ltd.

Chapter 5 · Nursing Care Of Patients Receiving Parenteral Nutrition

The total nursing care of patients receiving parenteral nutrition requires much consideration. Their problems are likely to be complex, and the management of parenteral nutrition will be only one aspect of their care. The responsibility of the nurse is to administer the feeding safely and with the least discomfort to the patient. The life of the catheter can be prolonged and the risk of complications minimized by meticulous care.

Care of the nutrient fluids

Parenteral nutrition fluids must not be administered to a patient until radiological examination has shown the catheter tip to be in a satisfactory position. Physiological saline can be infused, or a solution of heparinized saline injected into the catheter to keep it patent.

The preparation of fluids is undertaken by the pharmacy (Chapter 3) and should not, under any circumstances, be carried out in an unsterile ward area. Fat emulsions and solutions which have been mixed or contain additives must be stored at 4°C, ideally in a refrigerator solely for this purpose. Other solutions must be stored below 25°C and away from sunlight. An opaque cover placed over the container during storage and infusion prevents the degradation of nutrients by ultra violet light.

Fluids should be checked at the bedside by two nurses, one of whom must be qualified. A specific prescription sheet makes checking easier and safer. The prescription sheet should be compared with the label on the containers, paying attention to the expiry date. Containers should be inspected against the light for cracks and leaks, and for the presence of particles or cloudiness which would indicate contamination. They need to be checked regularly during infusion for signs of precipitation, which would indicate a delayed chemical interaction.

Preventing catheter-associated problems

Following insertion of a central line the patient needs to be monitored closely. The site of insertion should be observed for haemorrhage or leakage of fluid from beneath the dressing. If the subclavian route has been used, the patient should be watched for signs of a pneumothorax—chest pain, dyspnoea and cyanosis.

The main mechanical problems associated with central venous catheters are:

air embolism
catheter blockage
catheter fracture
catheter leakage

The risk of these happening can be reduced in the following ways:

1   Check regularly that the catheter is well secured to the patient.
2   Traction on the catheter can be prevented by applying a firm dressing to the catheter entry site and by securing a loop of the administration set to the patient using adhesive tape.
3   Administration sets with luer locks should be used, with their ends locked gently and securely together.
4   When the infusion system needs to be disconnected, the catheter should be occluded with a pair of atraumatic clamps. It is advisable to use a short extension tube between the catheter and administration set for clamping purposes, because frequent clamping of the catheter may fracture it.
5   Catheter blockage may be prevented by maintaining the flow of the infusion. It should never be turned off, as blood will clot within the catheter. If an intermittent infusion is required, e.g. at night time only, injecting the catheter with heparinized saline will keep it patent.
6   Attempts to relieve catheter blockage should not be made by inexperienced staff (p. 59).
7   Any leaks of fluid from the system need to be attended to

immediately. Administration sets must be renewed. No attempt should be made to stop leakage using adhesive tape.

Peripheral lines need to be well secured. They must be checked regularly for the common problems of thrombophlebitis and extravasation—pain, swelling and redness around the infusion site. Using a transparent dressing makes the site easier to observe.

Preventing infection

Nurses must be aware of the ways in which micro-organisms can enter the circulation. Protocol for handling the catheter and infusion system needs to be developed to prevent contamination occurring. It should be simple but effective, and must be adhered to rigidly. It should incorporate the following important points:

1 Thorough handwashing before touching any part of the system.

2 The catheter should be inserted in the cleanest possible environment using an aseptic technique.

3 Ensure that the catheter is used for feeding only—not for the giving or taking of blood, administration of drugs or measurement of central nervous pressure.

4 Addition to nutrient solutions should not be made in a ward area (but in a laminar-flow air cabinet by a trained pharmacist). If this is impossible, it is vital to work in a clean area, wear a mask and sterile gloves, and wipe bottle tops and injection ports with a suitable disinfectant.

5 The number of connections within the system should be minimal. This can be achieved by using;

    a) administration sets without injection ports

    b) single piece sets with two or three leads and Y connections, rather than multiple tap systems.

    c) administration sets with integral airways.

6) Administration sets should be changed every 24 hours with the fluid container.

7 Use an aseptic procedure when disconnecting the infusion system. Clean connections with a suitable disinfectant e.g. 0.5%

chlorhexadine in 70% spirit, and allow time for this to act. Wear sterile gloves when handling connections.

8   Care of the catheter entry site.

The dressing at the catheter entry site needs to be sterile and supportive, preventing movement of the catheter in and out of the insertion site. It should be comfortable for the patient. There has been much discussion about the most suitable types of dressing material to use. an occlusive, transparent membrane gives the advantage of a secure adhesive dressing. Occasionally, occlusive dressings cause irritation of the patient's skin. If a gauze dressing is preferred, it should be well secured to the skin with tape and it must be kept dry.

The actual dressing technique is probably more significant in keeping the infection rate low. Strict aseptic technique is vital. It is easier to dress a subclavian site if the catheter has been tunnelled away from the clavicle to an area lower down on the chest wall where it cannot be displaced by shoulder movements. The dressing may need to be changed one to three times weekly. If the administration set is plugged directly into the catheter hub, the dressing will need to be changed daily with the set.

Special Points:

a)   Sterile gloves and a mask should be worn for cleaning and redressing the catheter entry site.

b)   The skin around the catheter entry site should be inspected for redness and discharge, and a swab taken if these are found.

c)   The skin puncture site, catheter hub and surrounding skin is cleaned with a suitable antiseptic, e.g. 0.5% chlorhexidene in 70% spirit, or betadine alcoholic solution.

d)   If the catheter has been tunnelled, the original skin puncture site is also cleansed, and should be covered by a dressing until it has healed.

e)   An antifungal/antibacterial agent may be applied e.g. povidone iodine powder spray, before the dressing is renewed.

f)   If a transparent membrane is used, it is helpful to place a small piece of gauze over the catheter before applying the membrane. This prevents pulling on the catheter when the dressing is changed.

g)   If the catheter entry site is near the clavicle, it is helpful to apply the new dressing with the patient's head turned away from the catheter entry site and the shoulder abducted. It will then be less liable to subsequent displacement by shoulder movements.

Preventing metabolic complications

Many metabolic problems can be avoided by accurately controlling the infusion of parenteral nutrition, and by appropriate monitoring of the patient.

Accurate Flow Control

The flow rate should remain constant to ensure that the patient receives an adequate fluid and nutritional intake. A sudden alteration in rate may cause hypo or hyperglycaemia. Simultaneous infusion of fat emulsion with other solutions may be difficult, the low density of the fat emulsion may cause backflow. This can be overcome by positioning the bottle of fat at a higher level than the other containers.

Devices used to control flow rate are discussed in Chapter 4. An appropriate one should be chosen after considering the need for accuracy, safety, economy and ease of use. Nurses must be familiar with the equipment being used. It may be necessary to organise in-service training sessions to educate the staff. It should also be remembered that such devices are not a substitute for careful nursing.

Monitoring the patient

This is discussed in Chapter 7. Detailed nursing records need to be kept so that patients' progress can be assessed. Accuracy is essential because such records will influence the making of therapeutic decisions. A nurse spends more time with patients than any other member of the health care team so is likely to be the first person to notice change in a patient's condition. It is vital to be aware of the significance of any change, and to take appropriate action. Table

Table 5.1.

Temperature, pulse, respiration, blood pressure	4 hourly
Urine analysis for glucose and ketones	6 hourly
Fluid balance	daily
Nutrient intake	daily
Body weight — daily to assess changes in fluid balance	
— weekly to assess nutritional state	
24 hourly collection of urine for urea, creatinine and electrolytes	daily
Swabs from catheter puncture site for microbiology	as indicated
blood glucose measurements	as necessary

5.1 shows a checklist of the monitoring needed to be carried out by a nurse at the bedside.

Emotional Care

All those caring for parenterally-fed patients need to be aware of the problems which they are likely to face. A sensitive and understanding approach must be adopted, with attention to ways of boosting morale. A supportive family will be able to help a great deal.

Before the feeding starts, a simple description of the concepts of parenteral nutrition to the patient and family may help to alleviate some of the stress associated with it. A nurse assisting the catheter insertion can give reassurance to the patient.

A common problem is anxiety about the catheter and feeding system. Many patients become frightened when they realize how dependent upon it they are. They are liable to become distressed if any mechanical problems occur. It may be helpful to teach some patients about the care of their own equipment and about their daily monitoring.

Many factors may cause patients to be depressed—poor nutritional state and metabolic upset, surgery, gastrointestinal fistulae or a period in an intensive care unit. A patient who is acutely ill with gastro-intestinal disease will have no appetite or desire for food. However, some patients may find it difficult to adjust to the loss of such a basic function as eating. Days uninterrupted by meals may seem long and boring. The smell or sight of food may cause distress. Patients may feel isolated, especially if nursed in a single room. As their condition improves, they will benefit from exercise and a change of scene. The use of a battery-operated infusion pump or infusion at night-time only will give them more freedom.

Ending therapy

When the time comes for normal feeding to be re-introduced, patience and gentle encouragement is required. The dietitian needs to be involved.

Patients may have developed a heightened awareness of taste, especially of sweet food. Some complain of an uncomfortable feeling of abdominal fullness after eating. Small meals should be presented attractively, considering ways to tempt the appetite such as favourite home cooking or snacks between meals. If the patient is anorexic, temporary feeding with a fine bore tube may help.

The feeding catheter should remain in position until normal eating has been re-established. A record of the patient's food intake must be kept so that parenteral nutrition can be reduced appropriately.

Removal of the catheter

If the catheter has a dacron cuff, it will need to be dissected free in an operating theatre. Other types of catheter can be removed on the ward, using an aseptic technique. The patient lies with head downwards to prevent an air embolism. The catheter is withdrawn using a slow, steady pull, examined for completeness and its tip sent to microbiology for culture. A small firm, sterile dressing is placed over the exit site.

Home parenteral nutrition

A small number of patients will benefit from home parenteral nutrition. Such patients need to be suitably motivated, with satisfactory home conditions and family support. They will need to be carefully trained and supervised at a hospital base, which they should be able to contact at any time if problems occur.

THE ROLE OF A SPECIALIST NURSE

Some hospitals have found that employing a nurse specialized in the care of parenterally-fed patients has improved the overall standard of care.

Such a nurse can provide the following advantages:

1   Work as a member of a multidisciplinary nutrition team, advising on nutritional support for patients

2   Develop a nursing protocol with guidelines for all staff in the management of parenterally-fed patients

3   Educate and supervise staff caring for such patients. To be available for advice and for dealing with any problems which may occur

4   Participate in clinical development and research, which may involve the assessment of new equipment, monitoring the metabolic status of patients and collecting epidemiological data

5   Prepare patients for home parenteral nutrition, supervise and monitor them at home.

FURTHER READING

British Intravenous Therapy Association (1983) *Guidelines for the Nursing Care of Patients receiving Parenteral Nutrition*.

Davidson L (1986) Dressing Subclavian Catheters. *Nursing Times Nursing Mirror* **82**, 40.

Goode AW, Howard & Wood S (1985) *Clinical Nutrition and Dietetics for Nurses*.

McCanon L (1983) A Specialist Unit *Nursing Mirror* **156**, 50–1.

Morrow S (1982) Clinical Nurse Specialist in the Nutritional Therapy Team *Nursing Times* **78**, 1329–30.

Chapter 6 · Enteral Nutrition

Extra nutritional support is needed once it has become clear that a patient is unable to take adequate nutrition spontaneously from normal food. The ingestion of whole food, semi-solid food or liquids by the intestinal route is preferable to the more invasive procedures involved in parenteral nutrition. The type and extent of nutritional support necessary depends upon the patient's current ability to eat and drink, their clinical condition and the degree to which they were previously malnourished. In many patients with feeding problems one should not overlook the value of common sense; an encouraging chat and good food attractively presented may increase their calorie intake considerably.

Provision for individual food preferences can be difficult in the institutional setting, but an imaginative dietitian can usually modify the menu to meet the patient's particular likes. In some cases, introducing the family to the patient's nutritional problems and encouraging them to provide favourite foods which are otherwise unavailable is an added support.

The methods of providing nutritional support are considered in three sections:

    appetizing food high in calories and protein;
    semi solid or liquid food;
    tube feeding.

APPETIZING FOOD HIGH IN CALORIES AND PROTEIN

If a patient requiring nutritional support can tolerate whole food, then extra protein and calories can be given by providing calorie-condensed food including between-meal supplements. Some malnourished patients may have no appetite for a meal of meat and vegetables but with encouragement will eat breakfast cereals, sandwiches, soups, puddings, biscuits, cakes and sweets. Under-nourished patients should drink fluids which provide calories and protein; their customary water jug can be replaced by a jug of milk or milk shake. Alcohol (if not contra-indicated) can stimulate the appetite and provide additional calories.

Patients with feeding difficulties should be offered small quantities of food at frequent intervals. Daily food intakes should be recorded, and the approximate calorie and protein intake should be assessed by the dietitian, nurse or clinician using a simple check-list (Appendix pp. 259–61) or with the aid of food composition tables (Paul & Southgate 1978).

Table 6.1 summarizes practical advice which can be helpful for anorexic patients. There are many ways of adding extra protein and calories to ordinary food and liquids, the table on pp. 246–50 gives the nutritional content of some of the proprietary supplements currently available.

Table 6.1. Advice for patients to help overcome feeding difficulties experienced with a variety of conditions (e.g. gastrointestinal disease, cancer, especially during chemo or radiotherapy, immune deficiency states, motorneurone diseases)

Loss of appetite Feeling full too quickly	— Eat small, attractively presented meals—more often — Drink between meals rather than with a meal — Drink nutritious fluids, fruit juice, plain milk, milk shakes — Have an aperitif to stimulate your appetite — Avoid food rich in fat — Eat slowly and relax after a meal
Nausea and Vomiting	— Small frequent low fat meals — Try salty savoury foods rather than sweet ones — Eat dry foods such as crackers or toast — Try cool carbonated drinks sipped through a straw e.g. tonic water or ginger ale — Drink 30–60 mins before or after a meal — Let someone else prepare your meal
Mouth soreness and dryness	— Choose soft moist food — Avoid acid, salty and spicy food. Citrus fruit and tomatoes can sting or burn — Low acid fruits are better, bananas, pears, peach, apricot — Avoid hard dry foods which will scratch delicate tissue — Eat food warm and cold rather than hot — Ask for advice about mouth care

Table 6.1. *continued*

Feeling tired	— Use convenience foods, frozen meals and desserts, canned soups, milk puddings etc — Take regular rests — Accept offers of help from friends and family — Take nourishing drinks if you are too tired to eat e.g. Build-up or Complan
Change of taste	— If red meat is unappetizing eat chicken, turkey, eggs, and dairy products instead — Sharp foods may enhance flavours, e.g. orange or lemon juice, pickles, vinegar — Use herbs and spices in cooking — Try eating foods cold or at room temperature
Diarrhoea	— Eat foods low in dietary fibre, e.g. white bread, and cereals, use only cooked vegetables — Avoid fruit with tough skins and seeds, try banana or melon — Avoid fatty and highly spiced food — Drink plenty, eat little and often
Constipation	— Eat foods rich in dietary fibre, e.g. wholemeal bread and cereals, pulses, fruit and vegetables — Drink plenty of fluids, 6–8 cups daily — Hot fluids can stimulate the bowel, try hot lemon water first thing in the morning — Light exercise may help
Heartburn	— Eat smaller meals more often — Avoid fatty and highly spiced food — Don't lie down immediately after eating

SEMI-SOLID OR LIQUID FOOD

For those patients unable to take solid food, nutrient intake can drop dramatically unless an appetizing semi-solid or liquid diet with variety is offered. Liquidized hospital meals are often unappetizing and food of the same semi-solid consistency may be prepared in the form of fortified soups, light savoury or sweet egg dishes, flavoured sauces, savoury or sweet mousses, fortified milk-based puddings, or puréed fruit with cream. Too often a patient requiring a fluid diet is fed on clear fluids such as soup, tea, jelly and soft drinks instead of being given a planned feeding programme to provide optimum nutrition.

Palatability and variety are key factors: there are many proprietary specially formulated liquid preparations as well as those prepared in hospital which may be used as part of a fluid regimen. Some hospital-prepared fortified drinks are listed in Table 6.2.

Table 6.2.

Peachy milk shake 150 g tinned peaches 50 g skimmed milk powder 200 ml milk	25 g protein	435 kcal	375 ml
Cheap chocolate shake 50 g Complan 10 g drinking chocolate 250 ml milk	19 g protein	420 kcal	300 ml
Ambrosia shake 150 g tinned rice pudding 100 ml milk 50 g Polycal	9 g protein	390 kcal	300 ml
Orange juice 400 ml natural orange juice 100 g Polycose	3 g protein	532 kcal	450 ml
Tomato soup + caloreen 300 ml tinned tomato soup 50 g Caloreen	2.5 g protein	365 kcal	330 ml
High protein soup 200 ml tinned strained soup 50 ml milk 10 g Caloreen 15 g Maxipro	18 g protein	250 kcal	275 ml

Each recipe requires ingredients to be liquidized.

TUBE FEEDING

New apparatus and changes in attitude have given an impetus to tube-feeding practice. In the past, standard tube feeds, prepared in the hospital diet kitchen, were administered at intervals through a large bore Ryles tube which was passed into the stomach. More recently, feeds have been administered by gravity infusion or using enteral feeding pumps via a fine bore feeding-tube into the stomach or duodenum. The feeds usually used are ready prepared, commercial products. This section aims to summarize the materials and methods of tube feeding.

Feeds and their constituents

Many different feeds have developed over the years, both of the home-made and commercial variety. An old method still occasionally found is the use of normal hospital food, liquidized and syringed down a Ryles tube. With vitamin supplementation this, in theory, should provide adequate nutrition: however, the large quantities of fluid required to liquidize solid food often results in a volume of feed too large for the patient to tolerate and so the prescribed calorie intake is never reached. In addition, it is very difficult to calculate the composition of the feed accurately. In the past, hospital-prepared feeds have been made from mixtures of milk, eggs, cream, sugar and glucose; more recently, commercially prepared foods have been used (see Table 6.3).

Table 6.3.

Protein sources	Carbohydrate sources	Fat sources
Maxipro HBV (Scientific Hospital Supplies)	Maxijul (Scientific Hospital Supplies)	Calogen (Scientific Hospital Supplies)
Protifar (Cow and Gate)	Caloreen (Roussel)	Liquigen (Scientific Hospital Supplies)
Casilan (Farley)	Polycal (Cow and Gate)	
Skimmed Milk Powder	Polycose (Abbott)	
	Duocal (Scientific Hospital Supplies)	

See pp. 246–50 for nutritional composition.

Hospital-prepared feeds

Until recently many dietitians developed their own standard formulas based on proprietary products; minerals and vitamins were added according to the needs of the patient. A traditional hospital-prepared feed was a mixture of Complan and Caloreen.

Although the cost of a hospital-made feed is low, it is doubtful whether the patients' trace element and vitamin requirements are met during long-term feeding and osmolality is high. In addition, studies have shown that hospital-prepared feeds may become a source of bacterial infection and require regular microbiological monitoring (Anderton *et al.* 1986). Most hospitals, have turned to a commercially prepared ready-to-use feed.

Commercially-prepared ready-to-use feeds

A large number of commercially-prepared liquid and powdered formulas are now on the market (see pp. 239–45) varying greatly in composition and cost. They can be categorized into two main types. The majority are whole protein mixtures, containing protein, fat and carbohydrate in high molecular weight form and so have a relatively low osmolality: they require normal digestion. In contrast, the chemically defined products, often labelled 'elemental', contain amino acids alone or a mixture of short chain peptides and amino acids as the protein source, oligosaccharides and monosaccharides as the carbohydrate source, and fat mainly in the form of medium chain triglyceride. The nutrients are presented to the gut in a pre-digested form which aims to achieve maximal absorption.

The fixed composition of ready-to-use-feeds may sometimes limit their use in conditions which require modifications of a certain nutrient or electrolyte; the composition of a hospital-prepared feed can be designed to meet the requirements of the patient.

Formulating a tube feed

Protein

When gastrointestinal function is normal, adequate nutrition can almost always be achieved with feeds containing whole protein.

Most feeds contain milk protein but soya based feeds are available for patients intolerant of milk.

The products of protein digestion are absorbed in the form of peptides and free amino acids. Small peptides are absorbed more rapidly by the mucosa than the corresponding free amino acids (Silk 1974). The ad lib use of expensive elemental diets is waning and it is now accepted that their use may be justified in only a few conditions. A review of their composition, physiology and the indications for their use has been published (Koretz & Meyer 1980).

Elemental diets may be appropriate when the absorptive capacity of the intestine is greatly reduced or there is a shortage of digestive enzymes. Such diets can handicap nitrogen and calorie intake; they require slow introduction and can provoke reflux vomiting and gastric stasis (Jones *et al.* 1980a). They have a high osmolality and a rather unpalatable flavour and it is best to tube feed patients by continuous drip. Formulations containing protein mainly as short chain peptides are more palatable, lower in osmolality and are more acceptable physiologically (Silk *et al.* 1980).

The protein content of hospital-prepared feeds may be calculated to meet individual needs (p. 11). The non protein energy to nitrogen ratio of commercially-prepared feeds range from 100:1 to 200:1 which should cover the protein requirements of most patients.

Carbohydrate and fat

The common form of carbohydrate now used in both hospital-prepared and proprietary feeds is a polymer of glucose. The commercial preparations Caloreen, Maxijul, Polycose and Polycal are powdered starch hydrolysates low in free glucose with an average polymer length of 5 glucose molecules. They have the advantage of being only one-fifth the osmolality of glucose in solution and are virtually tasteless. The use of simple glucose as the carbohydrate source often precipitates diarrhoea. The lactose in milk-based feeds generally has an over-emphasized reputation for producing diarrhoea. There are however some groups for whom a lactose-free feed may be advisable. Patients with a damaged upper intestine, or those who have been undernourished may have a transient reduction in lactase activity. Also some Asian or African patients may have an inherited lactase deficiency.

The fat sources used in hospital-prepared feeds are Calogen a 50% emulsion of peanut oil and water or Duocal, a mixture of medium chain triglyceride, long chain triglyceride and glucose polymer. Proprietary complete feeds contain various vegetable oils. When problems arise with fat malabsorption, steatorrhoea may be overcome by substituting medium chain triglycerides (MCT) for long chain triglycerides (LCT). With a shorter chain length, MCT is partially soluble in water and can be absorbed more readily than LCT in the absence of bile or lipase. The chylomicron route of fat absorption is bypassed, and fatty acids derived from MCT are transported by the portal vein. Triosorbon and HiperNutril MCT are proprietary feeds with the majority of their fat present as MCT. Liquigen (50% emulsion of MCT and water) can be used in hospital-prepared feeds. In addition phospholipid and essential fatty acids must be supplied if MCT is the only fat source. The high osmolar load and rapid absorption of MCT may give gastrointestinal side-effects (e.g. nausea and diarrhoea). It is advisable to incorporate MCT into the diet gradually.

Vitamins and minerals

Vitamin and mineral requirements in disease are uncertain as pointed out in Chapter 1. Using current knowledge, the adequacy of the vitamin content of feeds must be checked. The table on pp. 239–45 includes the minimum volume of each feed required to provide the recommended intake of vitamins. There are many vitamin supplements available, documented in the *Monthly Index of Medical Specialities* (MIMS). Ketovite liquid and tablets (Paines & Byrne) together give the most comprehensive supplement, although Abidec (Parke-Davis) or Dalivit drops (Paines and Byrne) may be all that is required (pp. 236–7).

A feed with relatively low concentrations of sodium and potassium is more flexible; requirements for these electrolytes vary. Sodium and potassium supplements are easy to add in the form of their chloride salts. Additional trace elements can be given using Metabolic mineral mix or Seravit (Scientific Hospital Supplies) (pp. 237–8).

Osmolality

There are two expressions used to indicate the molar concentrations of a solute in a solution.
1 Osmolality—the number of osmotically active particles added to a kilogram of water;
2 Osmolarity—the number of osmotically active particles made up to a litre of solution with water.
Osmolality can be measured by freezing point depression and is a simple routine procedure in many hospital laboratories.

Ideally, a feed should have an osmolality close to that of plasma, 280–300 mosm/kg. This is best achieved if the feed is composed of whole protein, high molecular weight glucose polymers and long chain triglycerides. High osmolar loads tend to draw water into the gut lumen and cause diarrhoea. The lower the osmolality of the formula, the more rapidly the infusion may be given. However, Allison (1986) points out the importance of osmol administered per unit time rather than osmol per unit volume and describes how a patient is successfully fed overnight with a 1 litre feed of 2000 kcal with an osmolality of 420 mosmol/kg, using a constant infusion pump to maintain a slow and regular flow rate.

The total volume of feed prescribed for a patient normally dictates the calorie intake. The standard commercial feeds usually provide 1 kcal/ml. A calorie condensed feed giving more than 1 kcal/ml may have a relatively high osmolality and will therefore require slow infusion.

Water

Enough water must be given to accommodate the needs of renal excretion and to prevent the patient becoming dehydrated. A rough guide for an adult is 30 ml of fluid per kg body weight per 24 hours. If insufficient water is given hyperosmolar dehydration may result (Fowell *et al.* 1978). Care should be taken with feeds high in protein and electrolytes, especially in the young, the unconscious and the elderly and a fluid balance record should be kept.

Patients with head injuries may suffer cerebral oedema due to over hydration (Day & Buckell 1971).

Choice of feed

Standard feed

Hospital-prepared feeds can be made from supplements listed in Table 6.3, p. 78. Care must be taken in the preparation and storage of these feeds and a routine check for bacterial contamination should be made. Most centres prefer to use a commercially prepared feed, Fortison standard, Isocal, Clinifeed Favour, Ensure or Nutrauxil are good liquid formulas which may be used straight from the can or bottle. They are bacteriologically clean and can be stored unopened at room temperature.

Standard feed checklist

    Protein—Whole protein

    Energy—Glucose polymer, Fat

    Non protein kcal:N_2 ratio—150–200:1

    Osmolality—Isotonic with plasma

    Electrolyte content—Low

    Vitamins

    Trace elements

    Essential fatty acids

    Viscosity—Low

    Sterile—Free from contamination

    Cost—Low

Low protein, low sodium and potassium feeds

Low protein, low electrolyte feeds may be requested for intensive care patients or for patients in renal failure. Maxipro HBV is an excellent low electrolyte protein source, which can be supplemented with energy from carbohydrate (Polycose, Polycal, Caloreen or Maxijul) and fat (Calogen) or a combined energy source (Duocal).

Hospital-prepared feed

	Nutritional content:
45 g Maxipro HBV	protein 40 g
400 g Duocal powder	kcal 2040
25 g Seravit (minerals &	Na mmol 9.3
vitamins)	K mmol 5.5
Water to a volume of 2 litres	

The values of sodium and potassium are very low and supplements may be required to bring the values to the prescribed level.

Alternatively a commercially-prepared feed may be used for the protein and electrolyte source, e.g. Fortison low-sodium or Clinifeed Iso, with extra energy supplemented if necessary.

High protein high energy feeds

Tube feeds with a high protein and energy content can be formulated using a mixture of proprietary products or by supplementing a commercially prepared feed. Examples are given here.

Hospital-prepared feed

	Nutritional content:
1500 ml cow's milk	protein 110 g
330 g Complan	kcals 3560
200 g Caloreen	Na mmol 124
100 ml Calogen	K mmol 100
3 Ketovite tablets	
Water to a volume of 3 litres	

Commercially prepared feed

Ensure plus (62 g protein, 1500 kcal/1), Fortison Energy-Plus (50 g protein, 1500 kcal/1) and TwoCal HN (83 g protein, 2000 kcal/1) are ready-to-use commercial preparations which provide a high protein and energy content in a given volume.

Alternatively, a commercially prepared feed can be supplemented, e.g. Clinifeed Protein Rich is a liquid high protein feed. If instead of water a 25%, Caloreen solution is used to dilute the contents of each can to a volume of 500 ml, a 3 litre feed will

provide:

	Nutritional content:
6 cans Clinifeed Protein Rich	protein 180 g
+ 750 ml 25% Caloreen	kcals 3750
solution	Na mmol 80
3 litres total volume	K mmol 130

These large volumes of concentrated feed should only be administered by continuous drip feeding. Of the three major nutrients fat exerts the least osmotic load and is the most calorific; it is therefore a useful additive for high energy feeds. Patients with a normal gastrointestinal tract may tolerate up to 50% of their calories as fat.

All other factors considered, a palatable feed is an advantage as:
(a) regurgitation may occur in tube fed patients;
(b) the feed can be taken orally if necessary.

Administration

Choice of tube

There are a large variety of feeding tubes currently available, differing in length, material, bore and luer fitting (see Table 6.4). Tubes made of PVC tend to stiffen and become brittle after contact with gastric juice, ten days is the recommended length of time they should stay '*in situ*'. The polyurethane tubes are recommended for long-term use—up to six months.

Table 6.4.

	Material	Length cm	Gauge	Luer	Guidewire
Clinifeed (Roussel)	PVC	85	1 mm internal diameter	Male	✓
Prima tube (Portex)	PVC	85	6/8FG *	Male	✓
Silk unweighted	Polyurethane	92	6FG	Female	✓
Silk weighted	Polyurethane	92	6FG	Female	✓
Corsafe weighted (Merck)	Polyurethane	110	8FG	Female	✓
Fortison tube (Cow and Gate)	Siliconized PVC	85.5	1 mm/1.5 mm internal diameter	Male	✓
Vygon Code 2396	Silicone	90/125	6/9FG	Female	X
Viomedex standard	Polyurethane	110/140	9FG	Male	X
Viomedex fine line	Polyurethane	110	9FG	Male	X
Duo-Tube (Argyle)	Silicone	102	14/15FG	Female	X
Indwell (Argyle)	Polyurethane	91/107	5/8FG	Female	X

*FG (French gauge) = external circumference in mm.

Many of the more flexible tubes require a guide wire or stylet to stiffen the tube for insertion, the stylet is passed into the lumen of the tube prior to insertion and is then withdrawn once the tube is in place. Great care must be taken with this procedure to ensure that the stylet does not protrude through the distal end of the tube.

To ensure that a reservoir of nasogastric feed is not administered into a vein by mistake, some manufacturers have reversed the luers of their apparatus, putting a male luer on the feeding tube and a female luer on the giving set. An intravenous giving set normally has a male luer.

The PVC Ryles tube is still probably the most suitable for

unconscious patients. It is easy to pass, its position can be checked simply, and the stomach can be aspirated without difficulty to avoid the risks of inhaling stomach contents. In conscious patients a flexible fine bore tube is more comfortable, as it is easier for the patient to cough and swallow, and erosion of the nasal passage and oesophagus is prevented. The use of a fine bore tube necessitates the use of a continuous feeding technique as the size of the tube will not allow passage of large volumes of feed in a short time. If the patient is being encouraged to eat with a feeding tube in place, a fine bore tube should be used.

Procedure for nasogastric intubation

1 Provide privacy and explain the procedure and its purpose to the patient.
2 Place the patient in a sitting position with neck slightly flexed. Ensure the nostrils are clean.
3 Measure approximate length of tube required. For placement into the stomach measure the length from the tip of the nose to the earlobe and then from the earlobe to the xiphoid process. Add 50 cm to this length.
4 If a stylet is used, lubricate the stylet and insert into the feeding tube. Passage of a tube with a stylet should be carried out by an experienced nurse or qualified doctor.
5 Lubricate the tip of the tube and pass it posteriorly, ask the patient to swallow sips of water as the tube is passed.
6 Once the tube is beyond the nasopharynx, allow the patient to rest a little.
7 Ask the patient to swallow with neck flexed as the tube is advanced.
8 If the patient coughs or becomes cyanosed withdraw the tube to the nasopharynx and try again.
9 Remove stylet.
10 Confirm the tube is in the stomach by a) aspiration of gastric contents, b) by pushing air through the tube and listening with a stethoscope over the stomach or c) by X-ray.

11   Spiggot the tube and using non-allergic tape secure to the patient's nose in a comfortable place.

When any type of nasogastric feeding tube is passed placement must be checked. Many of the tubes are small enough to pass into the bronchial tree without interfering with respiration. Enteral solutions passed through a misplaced tube can cause death.

Care should be taken with silicone or polyurethane tubes passed without a stylet, they should be introduced slowly into the nostril otherwise they can kink and cause the patient to retch. Fine bore tubes can be passed under direct vision using a fibreoptic endoscope in patients with oesophageal or gastric strictures (Keohane *et al.* 1983).

Nasoenteric intubation

Nasoduodenal or nasojejunal feeding may be preferable in patients with delayed gastric emptying, increased risks of aspiration and for those who are immediately post operative. Intubation of the duodenum or jejunum is often difficult, a tube with a weighted tip should be used. Ideally, once the tube has reached the stomach, the patient is turned onto the right side so that peristalsis motion of the stomach will pass the tube into the duodenum. Metaclopramide given prior to weighted feeding tube insertion can aid the passage of the tube (Whatley *et al.* 1984). However peristalsis cannot be relied upon to pass the tube through the pylorus, especially in the typical post operative patient with gastric atony and/or dilatation, and endoscopic placement of the tube is often necessary (Keohane *et al.* 1983). Recently a procedure for nasoenteric intubation at the bedside has been described by Thurlow 1986, utilizing a method of corkscrewing the feeding tube to pass the pylorus.

Feeding enterostomies

The surgical insertion of a feeding tube or catheter into the gastrointestinal tract allows effective enteral nutritional support in patients for whom the nasoenteric route is unavailable. With certain diseases the upper gastrointestinal tract is obstructed but the small bowel and colon are intact, e.g. oesophageal stricture or tumor, gastric or duodenal tumor. With these conditions the operative insertion of a feeding tube distal to the lesion will allow normal digestion and absorption of food to take place.

Jejunostomy in particular is a valuable adjunct to gastric surgery and is probably the most common enterostomy performed. The recognition that small bowel function returns rapidly following surgery has stimulated the use of jejunostomies to enable early post operative feeding (Fairfull-Smith & Freeman 1980).

Details of surgical techniques for feeding enterostomies can be found in Rombeau and Caldwell 1984.

A standard isotonic feed is suitable for most patients with a gastrostomy or jejunostomy. Steatorrhoea in intrajejunal feeding may result from inadequate mixing of the food with bile and pancreatic juices; this may be overcome by using a formula in which the fat is predominantly MCT, or a formula which is low in fat and the protein is in the form of short chain peptides. Continuous drip or bolus feeding may be practised with a feeding gastrostomy, the jejunum cannot act as a reservoir for food and so continuous drip feeding is necessary for a feeding jejunostomy and regulation with a pump is often required.

Introduction and delivery of feed

The gradual introduction of full strength feed over a period of hours is recommended for most post-operative patients (see introduction regimen), rapid introduction can cause abdominal distension colicky pains as well as nausea and diarrhoea.

Gastric emptying must be established, particularly in unconscious patients, before a fine bore feeding tube is passed and a feed is given by continuous drip. If there is doubt about gastric emptying a Ryles tube should be passed and the following procedure practised.

Introduction regimen

> 30–60 ml water per hour for 4–8 hours aspirate after 4 hours.
> Little or no aspirate *then*
> 30–60 ml 1/2 strength feed per hour for 4–12 hours aspirate 4
> hourly.
> If absorption is satisfactory continue to strength feed volume
> prescribed aspirate 4 hourly.

Slow increase of volume and concentration of feed is important when introducing feed to a rested gut. For patients who have been taking some food by mouth a full strength isotonic feed may be used from day one. Once full strength feed is tolerated an intermittent feeding regimen may be followed or a fine bore tube can be passed and the feed administered by continuous drip.

The position of the tube must be checked at intervals, aspirations should be fairly regular at first and all patients should have the tube aspirated at least once during the night even when the feed is well established to ensure that the flat position in bed is not inhibiting gastric emptying. Regular aspiration is especially important for patients in intensive care, for the unconscious and those on drug therapy which may interfere with absorption. For example morphine and related drugs cause a decrease in gastrointestinal motility and can delay the passage of gastric contents through the duodenum for as much as 12 hours (Goodman & Gillman 1980).

Intermittent versus continuous feeding

For optimal nutrient intakes to be achieved, total volume of feed and method of delivery must be considered. The traditional intermittent method of delivery known as bolus feeding requires a nurse to pour a proportion of the total volume down the feeding tube at timed intervals. Volume per feed and number of feeds per day must be prescribed. Volumes exceeding 350 ml per feed may be poorly tolerated and when large volumes of total intake are required more frequent feeds are necessary.

An alternative method of feeding by continuous drip for a

period of 12–24 hours has helped to overcome some of the problems associated with bolus feeding (diarrhoea, nausea, vomiting, regurgitation, abdominal distension). Absorption is improved by slow delivery (Heketsweiler *et al.* 1975) and concentrated feeds are more likely to be tolerated. In addition it has been shown that with continuous infusion, nursing time is halved compared with the bolus method (Woolfson *et al.* 1976) and a more accurate fluid balance can be kept.

Patients may be fed continuously for a period during the night and then encouraged to eat during the day, or they may be fed during the day only or for a full 24 hours. A disadvantage of continuous drip feeding is that the patient is 'tied' to the apparatus during the infusion. Some manufacturers have overcome this by producing a carry pack which allows mobile patients much more freedom.

It is not known if one technique (intermittent or continuous) is physiologically better than the other in patients who require nutritional support. It has been suggested that a continuous infusion may be metabolically less efficient in the post-operative period however, Weir *et al.* 1986 failed to show an improvement in nitrogen balance when feed was administered intermittently.

Controlled prospective studies are needed to compare intermittent and continuous feeding with regard to nutrient utilization, body composition and hormone substrate interaction. A compromise which suits some patients well is to administer the feed by continuous drip for a short period followed by a rest for a similar length of time, over a period of 12–24 hours (see Fig 6.1).

There are several delivery systems available for administering feed by continuous drip, those currently available are marketed by Abbott laboratories, B Braun, Cow and Gate, Fresenius, Kabi-Vitrum, Portex, Roussel, Viomedex and Vygon.

The proprietary feeds Nutrauxil, Liquisorb, Fresubin, Nutricomp F and the Fortison range are marketed in bottles with accompanying giving sets so that feed is dripped from the bottle directly. The drip rate is difficult to regulate with some delivery systems and routine use of enteric feeding pumps has been proposed (Dobbie

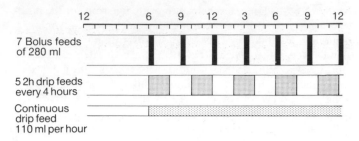

Fig. 6.1. Three Methods of giving a 2 litre feed.

& Hoffmeister 1976). These are expensive items and probably better reserved for patients who require close control of the infusion, e.g. intrajejunal feeding or who have gastrointestinal side-effects which don't respond to alteration of feed or medication (Jones *et al.* 1980b).

Monitoring

An accurate record of daily intake must be kept. Routine weighing and biochemical monitoring (Chapter 7) are essential in tube-fed patients. Initially, daily measurement of nitrogen output is necessary to estimate, nitrogen requirements. Once satisfactory feeding is established, twice weekly measurements are all that is necessary unless the clinical condition of the patient changes.

Enteral feeding must be established prior to the termination of parenteral feeding, daily communication between physician, pharmacist and dietitian will enable parenteral and enteral regimen to be dovetailed, phasing out the parenteral and increasing the enteral.

Complications

Diarrhoea is the major problem associated with nasogastric feeding and can be provoked by any of the following:

1 Bolus administration.
2 High osmolar feed.
3 Rapid introduction of full strength feed to a rested gut.
4 Antibiotic therapy (BMJ Editorial 1975).
5 Rapid gastric emptying, due to metoclopramide therapy.
6 Lactose intolerance.
7 Bacterial contamination of feed.

We have found the recommendation made by Woolfson *et al.* (1976) useful in controlling diarrhoea and add codeine phosphate syrup to the feed (30–150 mg daily).

Fluid and metabolic electrolyte abnormalities must be corrected where necessary by altering the volume or composition of the feed.

Home feeding and follow up

The majority of the commercial complete feeds are prescribable on FP 10 forms (Marked ACBS). The Advisory Committee on Borderline Substances list the conditions for which each product is prescribable in *MIMS*.

With careful instruction and supervision patients can tube-feed themselves at home, by continuous drip, for a full 24 hours or as an overnight feed.

Most patients who require extra nutritional support in hospital may still be underweight when discharged. Dietary advice should be given prior to discharge and close follow-up kept until the patient has a good nutritional status.

REFERENCES

Allison SP (1986) How I feed patients enterally. *Proceedings of the Nutrition Society*, **45**, 163–169.

Anderton A, Howard JP & Scott DW (1986) Microbiological control in enteral feeding. *Human Nutrition: Applied Nutrition*, **40A**, 163–7.

British Medical Journal (1975) *Editorial Antibiotic Diarrhoea*, **4**, 243–4.

Day S & Buckell M (1971) Feeding the unconscious patient. *Proc Nutr Soc*, **30**, 184–190.

Dobbie RP & Hoffmeister JA (1976) Continuous pump-tube enteric hyperalimentation. *Surg Gynaecol Obstet*, **143**, 273–6.

Fairfull-Smith RJ & Freeman JB (1980) Immediate post-operative enteral nutrition with a non-elemental diet. *J Surg Res*, **29**, 236–239.

Fowell E, Lee HA & Dickerson JWT (1978) *Nutrition in the Clinical Management of Disease*, pp 338–339, eds Dickerson JWT, Lee HA. Edward Arnold (Publishers) Ltd.

Goodman Gilman A, Goodman LS & Gilman A (1980) *Goodman and Gilman's The Pharmacological Basis of Therapeutics* 6th Edition. MacMillan Publishing Co Inc.

Hecketsweiler P, Vidon N & Bernier J (1975) Etude de l'absorption intestinale de deux solutions nutritives complexes au cours d'une perfusion intestinale a debit continu. *Reanimation Enterale (Les Colloques de l'Institut National de la Santé et de la Recherche Medicale)*. *INSERM*, 20 Nov 1975, **53**, 63–70.

Jones DC, Rich AJ, Wright PD & Johnson IDA (1980a) Comparison of proprietary elemental and whole-protein diets in unconscious patients with head injury. *Br Med J*, **1**, 1493–1495.

Jones BJM, Payne S & Silk DBA (1980b) Indications for pump-assisted enteral feeding. *Lancet*, **i**, 1057–1058.

Keohane PP, Attrill H & Silk DBA (1983) Endoscopic placement of fine bore nasogastric and nasoenteric feeding tubes. *Clin Nutr*, **1**, 245.

Koretz RL & Meyer JH (1980) Elemental diets—facts and fantasies. *Gastroenterology*, **78**, 393–410.

Paul AA & Southgate DAT (1978) *The Composition of Foods*, 4th ed. HMSO

Rombeau JL & Caldwell MD (1984) *Enteral and tube feeding*. WB Saunders Co.

Silk DBA (1974) Peptide absorption in man. *Gut*, **15**, 494–501.

Silk DBA, Fairclough PD, Clark ML, Hegarty JE, Marrs TC, Addison JM, Burston D, Clegg KM & Matthews DM (1980) Use of a peptide rather than free amino acid nitrogen source in chemically defined elemental diets. *J Parenteral Enteral Nutr*, **4**, 548–53.

Thurlow PM (1986) Bedside enteral feeding tube placement into duodenun and jejunum. *J Parenteral Enteral Nutr*, **10**, 104–5.

Wier A, Richardson RA, Carr K, Shenkin A, Garden OJ & Browning GG (1986) A comparison of continuous and intermittent post-operative naso-gastric nutrition after major head and neck surgery. *Proceedings of the Nutrition Society*, **45**, 74A.

Whatley K, Turner WW, Dey M, Leonard J & Guthrie M (1984) When does metoclopramide facilitate transpyloric intubation? *J Parenteral Enteral Nutr*, **8**, 679–681.

Woolfson AMJ, Ricketts CR, Hardy SM, Saour MD, Pollard BJ & Allison SP (1976) Prolonged naso-gastric tube feeding in critically ill and surgical patients. *Postgrad Med J*, **52**, 678–82.

Chapter 7 · Patient Monitoring

Successful monitoring prevents most of the complications associated with intensive nutritional support.

The frequency of each investigation depends upon the state of the patient's underlying disease, his response to feeding and the development of complications. As a general rule investigations need to be performed less frequently as nutrition becomes established and the patient's condition improves. Common sense and clinical judgement ensure that only the necessary investigations are performed.

If a patient has an intact gastrointestinal tract and is being fed enterally then monitoring is usually less frequent than with parenteral nutrition. If nutrition is being managed jointly between a nutrition team and the patient's own clinicians then there must be good coordination to ensure that any changes in the patient's condition are known to both and that all necessary investigations are being performed.

RECORDING INFORMATION

Accurate records are essential. They may be considered under three headings.

Normal ward charts

Temperature, pulse, blood pressure, etc.
Urinalysis chart—especially for glucose
Fluid balance chart—this also records the amount of nutrient solutions given.

A central record

This chart is particularly useful in ill patients; it groups the information obtained each day so that changes taking place gradually over a number of days can be quickly recognized. An example is given in Fig. 7.1.

Fig. 7.1. Example of a monitoring flow chart.

			Date
Regime	Parenteral vol	ml	
	Enteral vol	ml	
	Carbohydrate	kcal	
	Fat	kcal	
	Nitrogen	g	
	Sodium	mmol	
	Potassium	mmol	
Blood biochemistry	Sodium	mmol/l	
	Potassium	mmol/l	
	Chloride	mmol/l	
	Bicarbonate	mmol/l	
	Urea	mmol/l	
	Creatinine	μmol/l	
	Albumin	g/l	
	Bilirubin	μmol/l	
	AST	iu/l	
	Alk Phos	iu/l	
	Glucose	mmol/l	
Haem	Haemoglobin	g/dl	
	PCV	%	
	WBC	$\times 10^9$/l	
	Prothrombin time	sec	
Urine	Volume	l	
	Sodium	mmol/l	
	Potassium	mmol/l	
	Urea	mmol/l	
	Creatinine	mmol/l	
	Urea/24 hrs	mmol/24 h	
	Creat. clearance	ml/min	
	Glucose	%	

Fig. 7.1. *continued*

		Date	
Other losses	e.g. Nasogastric		
	Loss vol	l	
	Sodium	mmol/l	
	Potassium	mmol/l	
Balance	Fluid Total IN	ml	
	Total OUT	ml	
	Balance	ml	
	N Total OUT	g	
	Balance	g	
	Na Total OUT	mmol	
	Balance	mmol	
	K Total OUT	mmol	
	Balance	mmol	
	Body weight	Kg	

A food record chart

For particular patients on oral diet. The daily food intake is recorded either by the nurse, dietitian or the patient himself. The calculation of food intake is only meaningful if the quantity of each food has been carefully recorded (see Fig. 7.2).

The food record may be continued as an out-patient along with a weight chart to document the patient's nutritional progress.

ORGANIZING INFORMATION

Correct timing of samples

Samples for analysis should arrive at the laboratory early in the day; in particular 24-hour collections should finish in time for the morning laboratory analysis. This is essential if nitrogen, electrolyte and fluid balances are to be calculated (see below) so

Food record chart

NAME

WARD

DATE

Please record all food and drink . Give careful description of the type and quantity of food in handy measures e.g. slices, scoops, tablespoons, teaspoons, mls.

Breakfast	FOOD	QUANTITY EATEN	Miscellaneous e.g. sweets, fruit, etc.
Mid Morning			
Lunch	FOOD	QUANTITY EATEN	
Tea			
Supper	FOOD	QUANTITY EATEN	
Bedtime			
daily food intake		TOTAL	kcals protein g.

Fig 7.2. Example of a food record chart

that the prescription for the next 24-hour feed can be decided and the pharmacy informed.

Avoiding a hyperlipaemic sample

A lipid infusion should finish at least 6 hours before the blood samples are taken, otherwise the sample will be hyperlipaemic. If hyperlipaemia persists at 6 hours, evident by a milky plasma, then the lipid infusion should be discontinued. Artefacts which result from the analysis of hyperlipaemic serum include a falsely low sodium, and altered enzyme results.

Balance calculations

The organization of information to calculate fluid, sodium, potassium and nitrogen balance is invaluable in the sick patient and should not be omitted. The aim of a balance calculation is to amend in the subsequent 24 hours the excesses or deficits of the previous 24 hours.

Patient intake

This is obtained from the fluid balance chart and from the food record chart; the concentrations of nitrogen and electrolytes should have been recorded on the bottles of the nutrient solutions and also on the prescription chart.

Patient output

Water, electrolyte and nitrogen loss from the body can occur in several ways as described further below, under Clinical Monitoring.

The balance can thus be calculated:

	Water (ml)	Sodium (mmol)	Potassium (mmol)	Nitrogen (g)
Intake:				
Output:				

Balance = Intake − Output.

CLINICAL MONITORING

Attention is drawn here to particular aspects of bed-side monitoring associated with nutritional support, and a check list is given in Table 7.1.

Care of the feeding line

Good care of the feeding line is crucial and is considered in detail in Chapter 5.

Table 7.1. Monitoring check-list.

Monitoring	Suggested initial frequency *
Clinical monitoring	
Patient examination	daily
Temperature, pulse, respiration and blood pressure	4 hourly
Ward urine analysis	6 hourly
Fluid balance	daily
Nutrient intake	daily
Body weight	weekly
Laboratory monitoring	
Haematology	daily
Full blood count	
Prothrombin time	2 × weekly
Folate and B_{12}	as clinically indicated
Iron, transferrin, ferritin	as clinically indicated
Biochemistry	
Blood: urea and electrolytes, creatinine	daily
Glucose	daily or as indicated
Calcium and phosphate	3 × weekly
Liver function tests	2 × weekly
Magnesium, zinc, copper	weekly
Acid-base measurements	as clinically indicated
Urine: urea and electrolytes, creatinine (24 hr collection)	daily
Other fluids: electrolytes (timed collection)	as indicated
Bacteriology	
Parenteral catheter skin puncture site	3 × weekly
Blood culture	as indicated
Catheter tip culture	on removal

* This is a frequency appropriate for an ill patient; however it must be adapted to the individual patient and can be expected to decrease as the patient improves.

Detection and investigation of pyrexia

A serious complication of parenteral nutrition is infection of the central venous catheter. The recognition of this depends on 4-hourly measurements of the patient's temperature, pulse and respiration rates. When a fever is noticed the patient should be examined to check for wound and chest infections or deep venous thrombosis. A mid-stream specimen of urine should be obtained, microscoped and cultured. Blood cultures must also be taken. The possibility of hidden foci of infection such as intra-abdominal abscesses must be considered before the fever is attributed to the central venous catheter. If all possible causes of fever can be excluded or if there is a strong suspicion of an infected catheter, then it must be removed and its tip cultured. The patient should be vigorously treated with antibiotics and a central line should not be introduced at least until the patient has been afebrile for 24 hours.

Detection of glucose intolerance

A urinalysis chart with regular testing for glucose is required for all patients receiving intensive nutritional support (see later).

Collecting and measuring fluid output

Fluid loss can occur in several ways. The volumes of urine excreted, nasogastric aspirations, drain and fistula losses should be measured and sent for analysis (see laboratory monitoring). Insensible fluid loss must be allowed for when calculating fluid output. The normal insensible loss is approximately 500 ml per day, but this rises to a litre with a fever of 39°C. In addition, sweating may add up to a litre of fluid loss.

LABORATORY MONITORING

Laboratory monitoring is considered under the following headings:

    electrolyte balance
    nitrogen balance

glucose homeostasis
minerals and vitamins
nutritional status

The monitoring check list in Table 7.1 includes liver function tests, phosphate and tests for acid-base disorders: these items are considered further in the Metabolic Complications chapter.

Electrolyte balance

The urine sodium and potassium concentrations are subject to physiological control. These controls become modified in illness due to haemodynamic and hormonal changes; in particular there may be a reduced ability to excrete sodium. Regular measurement of urine sodium and potassium ion concentrations is required to quantitate the loss and also to help analyse an electrolyte disturbance.

In addition the measurement of blood and urine creatinine concentration allows the monitoring of creatinine clearance, which is a useful measure of renal function, provided an accurate urine collection has been made.

The electrolyte content of other fluid losses should be measured if the losses continue and are of significant volume.

Nitrogen balance

The nitrogen content of the feed should be known and ideally the nitrogen loss should be measured directly on urine, fistula and other fluid losses. However, the Kjeldahl technique for its estimation is unsuitable for routine use.

A reasonably accurate estimation of total nitrogen loss can be obtained by measurement of the *24-hour urine urea excretion* (Lee & Hartley 1975), using the formula:

urine urea (mmol/1) × 24 hr urine volume (litres) × 0.028 × 6/5
= nitrogen (grams/24 hr).

The 0.028 factor converts millimols of urea to grams of nitrogen and the extra factor 6/5, corrects for the finding that urea is approximately 5/6 of total urinary nitrogen loss. The rest consists of purines, ammonia, creatinine etc. which are less variable in their excretion.

Other nitrogen loss can be allowed for as necessary:

(a)   Skin and faeces—daily loss is about 1–1.5 g.

(b)   change in blood urea concentration (i.e. to account for urea not excreted in the urine):

24 hr change in blood urea (mmol/1) × total body water (litres) × 0.028 = nitrogen (g)

[total body water (litres) ≃ body-weight (kg) × 6/10]

This is about 1 g of nitrogen per mmol change in urea in a 60 kg person.

(c)   nitrogen loss of other fluids—an approximate allowance is 2 g/1.

(d)   loss from proteinuria or protein-losing enteropathy (6.25 g protein ≡ 1 g nitrogen).

Blood glucose control

Testing for glycosuria should be supplemented by measurement of blood glucose. In the absence of glycosuria, a daily blood glucose measurement is sufficient in the initial management of a patient receiving intensive nutritional support. If glycosuria occurs or if insulin is used, the blood glucose must be closely monitored.

The ward use of a reflectance meter with glucose-oxidase impregnated strips enables frequent assessment of blood glucose levels. It is advisable that there are regular checks to ensure this system is accurate; any markedly abnormal level should be confirmed by laboratory analysis. Some patients receiving high calorie glucose infusions require administered insulin. To some extent this insulin need can be diminished by giving some calories as lipid. It has been suggested that hypermetabolic patients may achieve improved nitrogen balance by the addition of insulin to their nutrition.

Frequent subcutaneous injections of insulin according to sliding scales can be inefficient and uncomfortable for the patient. Insulin infusion is preferred and is best administered via an adjustable syringe pump. This enables a straightforward system of variable dosage as described below.

Guidelines for continuous insulin infusion (Woolfson 1981)

As well as glucose, amino acids should be given, otherwise depletion of plasma proteins may occur. Preferably there should be total nutritional support to sustain the metabolically stimulating effects of insulin. It is important to remember insulin can deplete circulating phosphate and potassium. To allow for this, phosphate should be infused at 30 mmol/24 hours and potassium at 100 mmol/24 hours, or according to patient requirements. Connecting the insulin infusion to the same line as the intravenous glucose removes the possibility that the glucose may be discontinued while the insulin continues, and avoids the risk of hypoglycaemia. The aims is to maintain blood glucose between 7 and 10 mmol/1.

The usual insulin starting dose is 6 U/hr. This can be given, for example, by diluting 30 units of soluble insulin in 10 ml of normal saline, delivered at 2 ml/hr using an adjustable syringe pump. The dose is then adjusted according to the blood glucose, initially on hourly estimations, which are reduced in frequency as stability is achieved.

Table 7.2 gives the action to be taken according to the blood glucose measurements.

Table 7.2.

Blood glucose		Action
< 4 mmol/l		Slow by 1 ml/hr
4–6.9		Slow by 0.5 ml/hr
7–10.9		Same rate
11–15	If lower than last test	Same rate
	If higher than last test	Increase by 0.5 ml/hr
> 15	If lower than last test	Same rate
	If higher than last test	Increase by 1 ml/hr

If rate becomes 0.5 ml/hr or zero—halve concentration and restart at 0.5 ml/hr
If rate becomes 4.5 or 5 ml/hr—double concentration and restart at 2.5 ml/hr

It can be expected that most patients will achieve stabilization of the blood glucose level by about 9 hours after starting the insulin regime. If the blood glucose fails to fall, then it may be useful to reduce the glucose infusion, and then to increase it again to its previous rate within the next 24 hours.

Initially, hourly urine measurements should also be made. This establishes the relationship between blood and urine glucose concentrations and in most cases allows subsequent hourly monitoring by urine glucose tests alone, with occasional checks being made on the blood levels.

Minerals and vitamins

Mineral measurements

Measurements are usually available for calcium, phosphorus, magnesium, iron, copper and zinc. A low plasma level, although associated with deficiency of the mineral, may in fact be due to a decrease of the transport protein. The correction of total calcium for changes in albumin is well known:

$$\text{Measured calcium (mmol/l)} + \frac{40 - \text{albumin (grams/l)}}{40}$$
$$= \text{corrected calcium (mmol/l)}$$

Certain transport proteins, e.g. caeruloplasmin, are acute phase reactants and may be increased in acute illness. Such a rise in caeruloplasmin would further limit the ability of a plasma copper measurement to reflect a decrease in total body stores.

In general for the trace elements, assessment of plasma and urine concentrations is an imperfect guide to possible changes in tissue concentrations.

It may be necessary to measure concentrations not only in blood, but also in the urine and other major fluid losses. Some notes follow describing measurements of the individual minerals.

Phosphate

Low plasma and urine phosphate levels indicate deficiency, (p. 120).

Magnesium

Although, like potassium, this is a predominantly intracellular cation, reduction of plasma and urine levels are associated with magnesium deficiency.

Zinc

Plasma levels are reduced in deficiency but are an insensitive guide to body stores. The urinary zinc loss is increased in the hypermetabolic patient and may be 50–100 μmol/day or more. Losses in gastrointestinal fluids can also be significant and values of 150 μmol/l or more have been reported (Wollman *et al.* 1979). Direct measurements may be required in individual patients.

Copper

Predominant excretion is via the biliary tract. Again plasma levels are an insensitive guide. Increased urinary copper excretion may be observed, e.g. 5 μmol/day, and loss from external fistulae is usually less than 5 μmol/day (Kay 1981).

Vitamin measurements

The commonly available measurements are for folate, B_{12} and prothrombin time for vitamin K.

MONITORING OF NUTRITIONAL STATUS

The problems of obtaining objective, simple and reproducible clinical or laboratory measures of nutritional status have been discussed when considering the initial assessment of the patient in Chapter 1.

In assessing improvement in the patient, the same problems apply. Recordable changes reflect disease as well as nutritional status, and this particularly applies to short-term changes. Any change in body-weight usually reflects a change in total body water.

The records of nutritional intake, nitrogen balance and secondarily the body-weight, are the most useful contributors to the monitoring of nutritional status, taken in conjunction with the overall clinical impression.

REFERENCES

Kay RG (1981) Intravenous nutrition-trace metals. In *Nutrition and the Surgical Patient*, ed. Hill GH. Churchill Livingstone.

Lee HA & Hartley TF (1975) A method of determining daily nitrogen requirements. *Postgrad Med J*, **51**, 441–5.

Wolman SL, Anderson GH, Marliss EB, Jeejeebhoy KN (1979) Zinc in total parenteral nutrition, requirements and metabolic effects, *Gastroenterology*, **76**, 458–67.

Woolfson AMJ (1981) An improved method for blood glucose control during nutritional support. *J Parenteral Enteral Nutr*, **5**, 436–40.

Chapter 8 · Microcomputer Application in Nutrition

The calculation of individual feeding regimes can be a tedious process. The decreasing cost and increasing power and portability of microcomputer systems has lead to their increasing use in this area. The two main functions of the programmes available are regime planning and patient monitoring.

Regime planning

This is used to tailor requirements to the individual needs of the patient and is achieved by the use of algorithms and formulae. Two techniques of calculation have broad application.

Volume/Weight-based calculations

This method is favoured by many workers in planning nutritional regimes in neonates and children where volume load is the main limiting determinant. These programmes utilize standard recommendations for gestational age and body weight (Insley & Wood 1984) to calculate the required total composition of the nutritional regime and generate a formulation for the pharmacist to prepare. This application is advocated on the grounds of ease of use for the requesting doctor and time saved in preparation of the feeding solutions (Rich *et al*. 1982). An interesting approach has been described recently in which a choice of commerical formulations is suggested by the computer for a given set of requirements (Krasner & Marino 1985). The most suitable can then be chosen on the basis of clinical need or cost. However, cost savings may be offset by the need to stock an unnecessarily large range of feeding solutions. Realistically, TPN requirements in most patients may be met by a few standard formulations.

The inclusion of safety limits within the programmes, for

example preventing administration of magnesium until the seventh day of life and preventing nitrogen: calorie imbalance, may guard against the prescription of inappropriate regimes. Further sophistication is achieved by prompting the requesting doctor for clinical information which would alter volume, such as automatically restricting fluid in neonates with cardiac failure, and by making corrections based on laboratory data (McMahon 1984).

Energy/Weight-based calculations

This approach calculates energy and nitrogen requirements from body weight with appropriate allowances for increased needs due to sepsis or trauma. Fluid and electrolyte requirements are calculated and adjusted for situations of increased losses and may take into account measured plasma values and losses (Colley *et al.* 1985; Goggin & Hoskins 1985). Programmes of this type can be run on programmable pocket calculators allowing assessment at the bedside by the nutrition team (Colley *et al.* 1985).

Patient monitoring

Estimation of water and electrolyte requirements is extremely difficult and accurate monitoring is the best method of assessment. A significant proportion of patients receiving total parenteral nutrition are receiving other parenteral fluids or have organ failure. It is also important to note that many drug formulations, particularly the antibiotics, contain significant quantities of sodium and their administration can upset predicted calculations (Table 8.1).

Graphical display of balance data can allow early identification of trends which might lead to fluid and electrolyte abnormalities if uncorrected. This information can then be combined with clinical data to allow planning of TPN and fluid therapy.

Overall Patient monitoring

Nutrition is but one facet of the complex management of the

Table 8.1. Examples of several drugs which contain appreciable quantities of sodium.

Type	Preparation	Sodium content per typical dose
Oral	Gaviscon Liquid	6.3 mmol/10 ml
	Magnesium Trisil Mixture	6.3 mmol/10 ml
	Panadol Soluble	18 mmol/500 mg tablet
IV bolus	Ampicillin inj	1.47 mmol/500 mg
	Azlocillin inj	10.85 mmol/5 g
	Carbenicillin inj	27.1 mmol/5 g
	Penicillin G inj (unbuffered)	1.68 mmol/600 mg
	Penicillin G inj (buffered)	10.4 mmol/3 g
	Phenytoin inj	1.05 mmol/250 mg
	Thiopentone	11.0 mmol/2.5 g
IV infusions	Erythromycin in 250 ml N/Saline	38.5 mmol
	Sodium Fusidate 500 mg in 500 ml N/Saline	88.8 mmol

acutely ill patient. Nutritional data of the types described may be integrated with other details of the patient record and which in the future will be increasingly computer based. One attempt to relate nutritional data to other clinical information and outcome by use of the APACHE system has been described (Chong *et al.* 1986). It is to be expected that further integration of data in this manner will occur perhaps with the additional application of techniques of artificial intelligence and decision support. However, it is important that such developments are introduced into the clinical setting only following proper critical evaluation. To date, none of the programmes described in the literature have been tested in relation to their actual benefit to the patient. The claimed savings in time for the doctor and pharmacist may be sufficient justification for their use, but improved patient care cannot be assumed to automatically accrue.

Implementing a TPN programme

Writing programmes, however simple, is a time-consuming process. Given the number now available or in development most people will find a system to suit their needs ready written. Before choosing it is important to make a careful assessment of the requirement, to decide who will run the system, enter the data and respond to the results and to estimate expenditure, including running costs, and potential savings. Since such systems provide new facilities, in some cases planning for a change of future work practice might be required. Hardware requirements are not predictable but by current standards an IBM-PC compatible with hard disk and printer will be a common choice and should enable access to most of the best available software. Whatever the choice of software, it is most important that it is thoroughly tested *in situ* with all the personnel who will use it before it is finally implemented. Too many computer systems which look superficially attractive fail to match expectation because of inadequate evaluation and end up causing more and not less inefficiency.

REFERENCES

Chong RWS *et al.* (1986) Use of the APACHE II severity of disease classification to identify intensive care patients who would not benefit from total parenteral nutrition. *Lancet*, i, 1483–6.

Colley CM *et al.* (1985) Pocket computers: a new aid to nutritional support. *Br Med J*, **290**, 1403–1406.

Goggin MJ & Hoskins HT (1985) Management of parenteral nutrition aided by microcomputer. *Med Inform*, **10**, 5–12.

Insley J, Wood B (1984) *A paediatric Vade-Mecum*. 51–67. Lloyd-Luke, London.

Krasner JB & Marino PL (1985) An analytical approach to creation of parenteral feeding solutions: implementation on a microcomputer. *J Parenteral Enteral Nutr*, **9**, 226–9.

McMahon P (1984) Prescribing and formulating neonatal intravenous feeding solutions by microcomputer. *Arch Dis Child*, **59**, 548–52.

Rich DS *et al.* (1982) An evaluation of a microcomputer in reducing preparation time of paraenteral nutrition solutions. *J Parenteral Enteral Nutr*, **6**, 71–5.

Chapter 9 · Metabolic Complications of Parenteral Nutrition

The therapeutic advances of parenteral nutrition have been associated with an increasing awareness of the metabolic complications that can occur with its use. Long-term nutritional support has also brought our attention to a number of deficiency states which previously have seldom been seen in routine clinical practice. The complications particularly concern parenteral feeding, but some are also relevant to enteral feeding. A summary is given in Table 9.1.

Table 9.1. Metabolic complications of parenteral nutrition.

Complications with carbohydrate
  Problems of different carbohydrate preparations
  Hypoglycaemia
  Hyperglycaemia
  Hyperosmolar coma
  Respiratory distress
Complications with lipid
  Over infusion
  Acute reactions
  Impaired pulmonary function
  Depression of immunity
  Impaired utilization
  Use in liver disease
Complications with amino acid infusions
  Elevation of blood urea
  Hyperammonaemia
  Acid-base disturbance
  Hepatic encephalopathy
Acid-base disturbances
Hepatic toxicity
Essential fatty acid deficiency
Mineral and trace element deficiency
Vitamin deficiency

COMPLICATIONS WITH CARBOHYDRATE

A number of different simple carbohydrates have been considered for intravenous use.

Maltose has a low renal threshold and is lost in large amounts in the urine.

Fructose can predispose to lactic acidosis and hypophosphataemia. Most is converted to glucose in the liver prior to tissue metabolism. A small amount is lost in the urine.

Sorbitol is converted to fructose and has similar metabolic consequences; large amounts may be lost in the urine with resulting osmotic diuresis.

Ethanol may also predispose to lactic acidosis.

Intravenous preparations containing sorbitol, ethanol, or fructose are available. They are contraindicated whenever hepatic or renal impairment is suspected because of the risk of lactic acidosis (Wells & Smits 1978); they are also unsuitable for the hypermetabolic patient.

Glucose is the most popular carbohydrate source of energy in spite of its irritant effect on veins and that exogenous insulin may be required for its utilization. Impaired utilization occurs particularly in the very young, the old, in malnourished or septic patients and in diabetics.

COMPLICATIONS WITH GLUCOSE

Hypoglycaemia

There are rapid insulin responses to varying glucose loads, but after prolonged intravenous nutrition, inappropriate hyperinsulinism can result from excessive islet cell stimulation (Dudrick *et al.* 1972). If a high dose glucose infusion is suddenly stopped, hypoglycaemia may occur. Therefore, when parenteral feeding is to finish, the infusion should be gradually reduced over 24 hours. Similarly if the intravenous nutrition has to be suddenly stopped, it should be replaced with a 5 or 10% dextrose infusion for 24 hours or until the regime is restarted. This is particularly important during surgical operations to prevent the possibility of an unrecognized hypoglycaemia. The '3-litre bag' system reduces the risk of hypoglycaemia by spreading the glucose load over 24 hours.

Hyperglycaemia

Patients who are unable to utilize glucose may develop hyperglycaemia and glycosuria even with low rates of infusion. If hyperglycaemia occurs, prompt evaluation is necessary, the usual causes being too rapid infusion of the feeding solution or the development of stress or sepsis. The sudden appearance of hyperglycaemia in a patient previously tolerant of parenteral feeding suggests the possibility of sepsis and a thorough search should be made for a septic focus. A full description of the detection and treatment of hyperglycaemia is given on page 104.

Hyperglycaemic hyperosmolar coma

If hyperglycaemia persists untreated there is a risk of hyperosmolar non-ketotic coma (Dudrick *et al.* 1972). This condition has a high mortality and because it can present with symptoms of drowsiness, disorientation and coma may lead to a misdiagnosis of cerebrovascular accident.

The treatment involves:
1 Stop parenteral feeding
2 Transfer to the Intensive Care Unit (Dagget *et al.* 1979)
3 Correction of the hypertonic state. Great care must be taken with the use of hypotonic solutions, e.g. half strength normal saline or 2.5% dextrose, in order to avoid a rapid intracellular shift of fluid which can result in cerebral oedema.
4 Administration of low dose insulin infusion, e.g. 2 units of soluble insulin per hour given by continuous intravenous infusion.

Respiratory distress

A high carbohydrate regime increases carbon dioxide production and may even result in respiratory distress (Elwyn *et al.* 1981). Reduction of CO_2 production by replacing some carbohydrate with lipid can relieve this condition.

COMPLICATIONS WITH LIPID

Fat emulsions have increased their popularity since the introduction of the soyabean extract (Pelham *et al.* 1981). The poor reputation of the earlier cotton-seed oil derivatives were due to side-effects such as gastrointestinal upset, hepatosplenomegaly, coagulation defects and anaemia—known collectively as 'the fat overload syndrome'.

Although the 'fat overload syndrome' has occasionally been attributed to soya bean oil, the clinical features are not those observed with cotton-seed oil preparations. There have been but occasional reports of post-mortem evidence of lipid accumulation in patients who have received intravenous soya bean oil emulsions (Hessov *et al.* 1979).

Lipid infusions in premature infants may also result in fat accumulation in the lungs (Levene *et al.* 1980) and the need for careful attention to the infusion rate is particularly critical in this age group (Barson *et al.* 1980).

The maximum recommended rate of an infusion for an adult is 500 ml in 3–5 hours for 10% lipid emulsion and 500 ml in 5–7 hours for 20% lipid emulsion. The total volume per day should not exceed 30 ml/kg bodyweight of the 10%, or 15 ml/kg of the 20% preparation.

The side-effects that have been ascribed to lipid are:

Acute reactions. These are uncommon and transient, e.g. fever, shivering, backache.

Impaired pulmonary function. There may be minor effects of lipid on pulmonary function during the infusion especially if the plasma is hyperlipaemic (Järnberg *et al.* 1981).

Depression of immunity. There have been some reports that lipid may impair cell-mediated immunity and granulocyte function (Fischer 1980; Jarstrand *et al.* 1978); the clinical significance of these findings is not known.

Impaired utilization. Particularly in severely ill patients, it is important to ensure that lipid is successfully cleared from the blood stream. Persistant lipaemia 6 hours after the lipid infusion suggests impaired utilization. Before starting the infusion a blood sample should be taken and centrifuged, if the plasma is opalescent the infusion should be withheld.

Utilization in patients with liver disease. Caution is usually recommended in the presence of liver disease although available information is controversial. There are however reports of successful use of lipid in patients with poor hepatic function (Rössner 1981).

COMPLICATIONS WITH AMINO ACID INFUSIONS

A discussion of hydrolysates is not appropriate as these are no longer in use.

Elevation of blood urea

Slightly elevated blood urea levels commonly occur during parenteral feeding but normal levels are not usually exceeded if renal function is adequate. A continued rise in blood urea may be due to dehydration or unsuspected renal impairment.

Hyperammonaemia

Hyperammonaemia has been reported in neonates receiving parenteral feeding. Symptoms include drowsiness, twitching and seizures (Heird *et al.* 1972a). This complication can be prevented by administration of sufficient arginine in the feeding solution as this is essential for ammonia metabolism in the urea cycle.

Hyperammonaemia may also occur in patients with liver disease.

Acid base disturbance

See below.

Hepatic encephalopathy

See Chapter 14.

ACID-BASE DISTURBANCES

Patients receiving intravenous feeding are liable to all the common abnormalities of acid-base homeostasis. The possibility of certain carbohydrate solutions causing lactic acidosis has already been referred to.

The main disturbance caused by parenteral feeding is hyperchloraemic metabolic acidosis, especially in patients with renal impairment. This tendency is due to:

1 The metabolism of cationic amino acid with the release of free hydrogen ions (Heird *et al.* 1972b).

2 The presence of an excess chloride load in some feeding regimes which may restrict the ability of the kidney to excrete hydrogen ion (Grant 1980).

3 The measured titratable acidity in some feeding solutions.

The prevention and treatment of such hyperchloraemic acidosis consists of reducing the chloride load by exchanging a proportion of chloride for acetate. Each acetate anion consumes a hydrogen ion when it is metabolized.

HEPATIC TOXICITY

Increases in serum enzymes of hepatic origin are not infrequently seen in patients receiving parenteral nutrition. The significance of these changes is unclear as in most cases enzymes return to normal after parenteral feeding has finished. Furthermore, many different factors such as sepsis and malnutrition may contribute to hepatic disturbance in these patients.

Most reports of hepatic toxicity have concerned fat-free parenteral nutrition (Macfadyen *et al.* 1979; Lindor *et al.* 1979; Sheldon *et al.* 1978) although it is likely that similar changes may occur if the feeding includes a triglyceride emulsion. Elevated hepatic enzymes have been reported also with nasogastric feeding (Tweedle *et al.* 1979).

There is a characteristic pattern to these enzyme changes. Transaminases may rise two or three fold about 8 days after the beginning of feeding. A similar rise in alkaline phosphatase may occur and may persist for longer than the transaminase changes. The elevation of alkaline phosphatase may be associated with a rise in bilirubin levels and even frank jaundice.

The causes of these changes are so far unknown. In part they may result from enzyme adaption to the feeding; but may be due to inadequacy of the feeding regime. Available biopsy reports have suggested a pattern of fatty deposition with possible progression to more chronic choleostatic changes.

The following approach to abnormal liver function tests should be made:

1   Exclusion of other causes of abnormal liver function:

2   If the changes in the liver function tests are moderate and correspond to the above pattern, then feeding can be continued with caution

3   If large and rapid changes occur, or if jaundice supervenes, feeding should be stopped to identify the cause.

It has been suggested that providing excess carbohydrate may lead to fat accumulation in the liver and that increasing the ratio of amino acids to carbohydrate may prevent such changes (Macfadyen *et al.* 1979).

ESSENTIAL FATTY ACID DEFICIENCY

There have been reports of essential fatty acid deficiency with lipid-free parenteral feeding (Riella *et al.* 1975) and also with enteral feeding (Farthing *et al.* 1980). Biochemical changes may occur 1–3 weeks after dietary deprivation and clinical deficiency can become evident soon after. Manifestations of deficiency include scaly dermatitis, alopecia, hepatomegly and thrombocytopaenia (Pelham 1981). For treatment see p. 30.

MINERAL AND TRACE ELEMENT DEFICIENCY

Phosphate

Extra nutritional support increases the cellular need for phosphate, and so depletes circulating phosphate. Hypophosphataemia usually becomes evident 2–4 days after starting feeding unless phosphate is provided (Knochel 1977). Symptoms usually do not occur until plasma phosphate falls below 0.35 mmol/1, when anorexia, weakness, bone pain and joint stiffness may ensue. Further symptoms include muscle weakness, tremor, paraesthesiae, confusion and coma as well as haemolysis and abnormal leukocyte function (*Lancet* editorial 1981).

There may be risks of excess phosphate administration. Care should be taken in the presence of hypercalcaemia as there is a risk of metastatic clacification. A regime giving 50 mmol of phosphate a day has been implicated in a bone disease occuring after long term parenteral nutrition. (Allam *et al.* 1980).

Magnesium

Deficiency can occur within a week of starting parenteral feeding, especially in patients with pre-existing depletion due to intestinal or renal losses. Muscle weakness, fasciculation, tetany, vertigo and depression are characteristic symptoms. Trousseau's sign may be positive and ST depression with T wave inversion may be seen on the ECG.

If deficiency has to be rapidly corrected then 40 ml of 10% magnesium sulphate (17 mmol) should be given as an infusion over 30 minutes.

Zinc

Deficiency is characterized by skin rashes, hair loss, diarrhoea, impaired olfactory and taste sensation, poor wound healing and depression (Wolman *et al.* 1979). Symptoms may already be evident within two weeks of starting zinc deficient parenteral nutrition.

Copper

Symptoms may take some weeks to appear. They include hypochromic anaemia, neutropaenia and osteoporosis (Lowry *et al.* 1977).

Other trace elements

Some 15 trace elements are now thought to be essential, mainly acting as co-factors in various enzyme systems (Aggett 1979).

Deficiency states of nickel, vanadium, silicon, fluorine and tin have been observed in experimental animals but not observed in man. Documented deficiencies in man are of chromium (Jeejeebhoy *et al.* 1977), selenium (Young 1981) and manganese.

Deficiencies should be avoided by the addition of trace elements to all the feeding regimes especially in long-term parenteral nutrition.

VITAMIN DEFICIENCY

The importance of vitamin supplementation has been stressed elsewhere in the book. The clinical effects of deficiency of vitamin B_1 (Nadel & Burger 1976), biotin (Mock *et al.* 1981), folate (Woods 1980) and vitamin C (Robson *et al.* 1980) have all been described during deficient intravenous feeding.

Acute folate deficiency has been reported during parenteral nutrition with the precipitation of life-threatening pancytopaenia. There is evidence that infusion of the amino acid methionine may be responsible by depleting available folate (Woods 1981). The provision of folate in the presence of B_{12} deficiency can precipitate the neuropathy associated with pernicious anaemia. Hence, prior to folate and B_{12} supplementation, B_{12} levels should be estimated so that a diagnosis of pernicious anaemia is not overlooked.

122   *Chapter 9*

REFERENCES

Aggett PH (1979) Trace elements in medicine. *Hospital Update*,5, 981–94.

Allam BF, Dryburgh FJ & Shenkin A (1981) Metabolic bone disease during parenteral nutrition. *Lancet*, i, 385.

Barson AJ (1980) *Safety of Intralipid. Lancet*, ii, 1021.

Daggett P, Deanfield J, Moss F & Reynolds D (1979) Severe hypernatraemia in adults. *BMJ*, 1, 1177–1180.

Dudrick SJ, Macfadyen BV, Van Buren CT, Ruberg RL & Maynard AT (1972) Parenteral hyperalimentation, metabolic problems and solutions. *Ann Surg*, 176, 259–264.

Elwyn DH, Askanazi J, Kinney JM & Gump FE (1981) Kinetics of energy substrates. 2nd European Congress on Parenteral and Enteral Nutrition. September 1980 Ed. Wright PD, *Acta Chir Scand Suppl*, 507, 209–19.

Farthing MJG, Jarrett EB, Williams G & Crawford MA (1980) Essential fatty acid deficiency after prolonged treatment with elemental diet. *Lancet*, ii, 1088–9.

Fischer GW, Hunter KW, Wilson SR & Mease AD (1980) Diminished bacterial defences with intralipid. *Lancet*, ii, 819–20.

Grant J (1980) Handbook of total parenteral nutrition, p 142. Philadelphia Saunders.

Heird WC, Nicholson JF, Driscoll JM, Schullinger JN & Winters RW (1972a) Hyperammonemia resulting from intravenous alimentation using a mixture of synthetic L-amino acids. A preliminary report. *Journal of Pediatrics*, 81, 162–5.

Heird WC, Dell RB, Driscoll JM, Grebin B & Winters RW (1972b) Metabolic acidosis resulting from intravenous alimentation mixtures containing synthetic amino acids. *New Engl J Med*, 287, 943–948.

Hessov I, Melsen F & Haug A (1979) Postmortem Findings in three patients treated with intravenous fat emulsions. *Arch Surg*, 114, 66–68.

Järnberg PO, Lindholm M & Eklund J, (1981) Lipid Infusion in critically ill patients. Acute effects on haemodynamic and pulmonary gas exchange. *Critical Care Medicine*, 9, 27–31.

Jarstrand C, Berghem L & Lahnborg G (1978) Human granulocyte and Reticuloendothelial system function during intralipid infusion. *J Parenteral Enteral Nutr*, 2, 663–670.

Jeejeebhoy KN, Chu RC, Marliss EB, Greenberg GR & Bruce-Robertson A (1977) Chromium deficiency, glucose intolerance and neuropathy reversed by chromium supplementation, in a patient receiving long-term total parenteral nutrition. *Am J Clin Nut*, 30, 531–538.

Knochel JP (1977) The Pathophysiology and Clinical characteristics of Severe Hypophosphatemia. *Arch Intern Med*, 137, 203–220.

Lancet Editorial (1981) Treatment of severe hypophosphataemia. *Lancet*, ii, 734.

Levene MI, Wigglesworth JS, Desai R (1980) Pulmonary fat accumulation after intralipid infusion in the pre-term infant. *Lancet*, ii, 815–818.

Lindor KD, Fleming R, Abrams A. Hirschkorn MA (1979) Liver function values in adults receiving total parenteral nutrition. *J Am Med Ass*, 241, 2398–2400.

Lowry SF, Goodgame JT, Smith JC, Maher MM, Makuch RW, Henkin RI, Brennan MR (1979) Abnormalities of Zinc and Copper during total parenteral nutrition. *Ann Surg*, **189**, 120–128.

MacFayden BV, Dudrick SJ, Baquero G, Gum ET (1979) Clinical and Biological Changes in Liver function during Intravenous Hyperalimentation. *J Parenteral Enteral Nutr*, **3**, 438–443.

Mock DM, de Lorimer AA, Liebman WM, Sweetman L, Baker H (1981) Biotin deficiency: an unusual complication of parenteral alimentation. *N Engl J Med*, **304**, 820–823.

Nadel AM, Burger PC (1976) Wernicke Encephalopathy Following prolonged Intravenous Therapy. *JAMA*, **235**, 2403–2405.

Pelham LD (1981) Rational use of intravenous fat emulsions. *Am J Hosp Pharm*, **38**, 198–208.

Riella MC, Broviac JW, Wells M, Scribner BH (1975) Essential fatty acid deficiency in Human adults during total parenteral nutrition. *Ann Intern Med*, **83**, 786–789.

Robson JRK, Vanderveen T, Bennett K, Thomson T (1980) Ascorbic acid deficiency during TPN. *J Parenteral Enteral Nutr*, **4**, 518.

Rössner S (1981) The relation of intravenous fat solutions to Lipoprotein metabolism. 2nd European Congress on Parenteral and Enteral nutrition. September 1980, Ed. Wright PD. *Acta Chir Scand.* Suppl **507**, p. 220–225.

Sheldon GF, Peterson SR, Sanders R (1978) Hepatic dysfunction during hyperalimentation. *Arch Surg*, **113**, 504–508.

Tweedle DEF, Skidmore FD, Gleave EN, Knass DA & Gowland E (1979) Nutritional support for patients undergoing surgery for cancer of the head and neck. *Research and Clinical Forums*, **1**, No 1, 59–65.

Wells FE & Smits BJ (1978) Utilization and metabolic effects of a solution of amino acids, sorbitol and ethanol in parenteral nutrition. *Am J Clin Nutr*, **31**, 442–450.

Wolman SL, Anderson GH, Marliss EB & Jeejeebhoy KN (1979) Zinc in total parenteral nutrition, Requirements and metabolic effects. *Gastroenterology*, **76**, 458–467.

Woods HF (1980) Metabolic complications with special reference to folate deficiency. *Topics in Gastroenterology*, **8**, Ed. Truelove SC, Kennedy HJ. Blackwell Scientific Publications pp. 51–62.

Young VR (1981) Selenium: A case for its Essentiality in man. *N Engl J Med*, **304**, 1228–1230.

Chapter 10 · Immunological Effects of Malnutrition

Clinical data from patients with protein-calorie malnutrition show an association between malnutrition and immuno-suppression even in the absence of infection.

The immune system can be considered in three broad groupings: humoral immunity, cell-mediated immunity and non-specific immunity, and Table 10.1 is arranged accordingly.

There are other possible factors that can modify the immune response, in particular infection and also trauma or surgery. Hence Table 10.1 indicates where these different aetiological factors may apply.

Cell-mediated immunity

The most striking findings relating to malnutrition occur in cell-mediated immunity, i.e. T cell mechanisms. The lymphocytes in peripheral blood are mainly T cells (65–85%) and a lymphocyte count reflects the approximate numbers of circulating T cells. The production of antibodies, especially IgG antibodies, to T-dependent antigens is also reduced, probably as a result of deficient T cell (especially helper T cell) and macrophage functions. The loss of Natural Killer (NK) cell activity may be associated with the failure to produce α- interferon.

The effects on cell-mediated immunity are nevertheless not specific for malnutrition. T cell functions, including skin tests, and T cell numbers can also be affected by trauma, and the abnormalities may persist for several months.

Humoral immunity

Measurements of total immunoglobulins are imprecise, but do reveal differences in IgG levels in gross malnutrition. Serial

124

measurements must be made on individual patients in order to be meaningful. The IgG response to individual antigens, such as vaccines, shows better correlation with malnutrition—however, live vaccines should not be used, especially oral vaccines since reduced mucosal immunity can result in systemic spread.

Non-Specific immunity

Some components of complement are reduced in association with malnutrition; these components are synthesized in the liver and reduced synthesis may be responsible for low levels in the absence of infection. Estimations of individual complement components may be more promising as nutritional markers and are simple to do. Measurements of C3 and C4 in serum are routinely available. Interpretation of neutrophil function tests is impossible if infection is suspected.

Summary

It is clear that although the immune response is susceptible to malnutrition, the complexity of the response and the interplay with other factors, such as raised plasma cortisol levels, do not readily enable these measurements to be used as clear-cut markers of nutritional status. Furthermore the effects of vitamin or trace element deficiencies on the immune system, though important, are unclear.

REFERENCES

Chandra RK (1983) Nutrition, Immunity and Infection: Present Knowledge and Future Directions. *Lancet*, **i**, 688–691.

Cunningham-Rundles S (1982) Effects of Nutritional Status on Immunological Function. *Am J Clin Nutr*, **35**, 1202–1210.

Dowd PS & Heatley RV (1984) Influence of undernutrition on immunity. *Clin Sci*, **66**, 241–8.

Table 10.1.

Test	Ease[1]	PCM[2]	Infection[3]
Humoral Immunity			
Total IgG in serum	R	↓[G]	↑
Total IgA in serum	R	N	N or ↑
Total IgM in serum	R	N	↑
Secretory IgA	S	↓	↓
Antibody affinity	C	↓	?
Cell Mediated Immunity			
Lymphocyte count	R	↓	↑↓
T cell count	R	↓↓	↑↓
Helper T cells (T4)	S	↓↓	↓↑
Suppressor T cells (T8)	S	N	↑
PHA transformation response	C	↓↓	N
Macrophage migration inhibition			
factor production	C	↓	?
γ interferon production	C	↓	↑
Skin tests: recall antigens: *Candida*	S	↓↓	?
: PPD[a]	R	↓	?
Primary sensitization (DNCB)[b]	S	↓	?
Non-Specific Immunity			
Complement:			
Total haemolytic complement (CH_{50})	R	↓↓	N
C3 C9	R	↓↓	↑
Factor B	R	↓↓	N
C3 Breakdown products	R	absent	present
C4 C5 C1	R	N	N or ↑
Neutrophils:			
Neutrophil chemotaxis	S	↓	↓↓
NBT test[c]	R	N	↑
Stimulated NBT test	R	↓	—
Intracellular killing—bacteria + fungi	R	↓↓	↑↓

Notes

1 East of test R = Routine

            S = Simple

            C = Complex

2 Findings in protein calorie malnutrition

        ↓ = reduced

        ↓↓ = markedly reduced

        N = normal

Table 10.1. *continued*

Species[4]	Reversal[5]	Useful
man	✓	Yes, in absence of infection
man	—	No
man	—	No
man	?	Yes—as response to oral vaccine
man	?	Limited investigation so far and complex procedure
man	slow	Also ↓ following surgery and trauma;
man	slow	limited value
man	✓	
man	✓	
man	slow	
man + g. pigs	?	Also ↓ following surgery and trauma and effects may
man	?	persist for several months despite clinical recovery
man	?	
man	?	
man	?	
man	✓	
man	✓	
man	✓	May be helpful
man	✓	
man	—	
dogs + man	dogs	
man	✓	May be helpful in absence of infection
man	✓	
man	✓	

3 Changes seen in infection

4 Species in which effect demonstrated—usually in man but if human data is scanty, animal work included.

5 Reversal by parenteral feeding if known

6 Based on few patients in whom no evidence of infection
   a PPD ° Purified protein derivative of tuberculin
   b DNCB ° Di-nitro-chloro-benzine
   c NBT ° Nitro blue tetrazolium

Chapter 11 · Bowel Rest in Inflammatory Bowel Disease

BACKGROUND

The concept of 'resting' the bowel as part of the treatment of inflammatory bowel disease is an old one. In 1913, J.Y. Brown of St Louis in the United States described the use of terminal ileostomy in the treatment of severe ulcerative colitis; thus providing physiological rest for the diseased colon. Unfortunately, it was found that it was seldom possible to restore the continuity of the bowel without recrudescence of the disease (Cattell 1948).

A similar approach has been tried in the treatment of Crohn's disease. Two groups of workers have performed by-pass operations for ileal or ileo-caecal disease (Koudahl *et al.* 1974; Homan & Dineen 1978). These operations were followed by persistent or recurrent inflammation in a high percentage of cases. However, workers in Oxford have reported encouraging results with the use of split ileostomy to divert the faecal stream in patients suffering from Crohn's disease of the colon (Harper *et al.* 1983).

This procedure has met with less success in some other centres (Jones *et al.* 1966; Oberhelman *et al.* 1968).

Renewed interest in the concept of bowel rest as part of the treatment of inflammatory bowel disease was aroused by the advent of elemental diets and parenteral nutrition (Winitz *et al.* 1970; Dudrick & Ruberg 1971). Bowel rest brought about by these nutritional methods avoids the complications of surgery and abnormalities, such as bacterial overgrowth in isolated segments, cannot occur. In addition, this approach provides good nutrition to patients who are frequently poorly nourished because of poor appetite, abdominal pain or partial intestinal obstruction resulting from their disease.

ENTERAL NUTRITION

The details of chemically defined or elemental diets are discussed elsewhere in this book (chapter 6). A diet of this type made up of monosaccharides, amino acids, electrolytes, trace elements and vitamins given for long periods was found to maintain normal nutrition in man (Winitz *et al.* 1970). The stool output is markedly reduced in patients taking an elemental diet and, in a study using ileostomists, Hill *et al.* (1976) found that the outputs of fluid, sodium, trypsin and bile acids through the ileostomy were all significantly reduced. Silk (1974) reported that it might be preferable to use oligopeptides rather than amino acids as these reduce the high osmolarity of the diet. Amongst others, O'Morain *et al.* (1984) have reported favourable results with the use of an elemental diet in the treatment of patients with Crohn's disease. In addition, these diets may be helpful as part of the treatment in patients with fistulae or severe perineal disease as a reduction in faecal volume may be beneficial. However, it is not certain whether this improvement occurs because of improved nutrition, or bowel rest, or a combination of both of these.

PARENTERAL NUTRITION

The use of parenteral nutrition removes the influence of food in the gastrointestinal tract. The presence of food in the intestine increases its motility, blood flow and mucosal cell turnover. In addition, it stimulates the secretion of fluid, electrolytes, enzymes, hormones and bile. Dudrick *et al.* (1976) suggested that the total bowel rest provided by parenteral nutrition might encourage repair of the damaged intestine. Several studies have shown that active Crohn's disease may enter remission in patients treated by parenteral nutrition and total bowel rest (Reilly *et al.* 1976; Mullen *et al.* 1978). This occurred in some patients with Crohn's disease of the small bowel, with or without fistulae, and in some patients with Crohn's disease of the colon.

Parenteral nutrition and total bowel rest have been shown to maintain the nutritional state of patients with severe ulcerative colitis, but the short-term prognosis and severity of the disease were not altered (Reilly *et al.* 1976; Mullen *et al.* 1978). However, 60% of patients with an acute attack of ulcerative colitis have been shown to achieve a remission of symptoms with a five-day course of intravenous steroids accompanied by partial parenteral nutrition (Truelove *et al.* 1978). Nevertheless, it is likely that the intravenous steroid therapy plays the major role in inducing remission in these circumstances. Giving the necessary quantity of intravenous steroids together with full parenteral nutrition may cause a high blood sugar in these patients. However if the standard regime with fat recommended on p. 39 is used these complications can usually be avoided.

All of these studies of parenteral nutrition and bowel rest that have been mentioned were uncontrolled trials. In 1980, Dickinson and his colleagues reported their results of a prospective controlled trial of parenteral nutrition and total bowel rest as an adjunct to the routine therapy of acute colitis. They found that the nutritional status was maintained in the group of patients receiving parenteral nutrition, as opposed to a marked loss of body protein in the control group. However, there was no significant difference in the frequency of surgery or the duration of medical treatment between the two groups. Weser (1980) has pointed out several deficiencies in this trial. The overall number of patients was small, the patients with ulcerative colitis and those with Crohn's disease were studied together, and the patients in the two groups were not well matched for the type or the duration of the disease. Further controlled studies of both elemental diets and parenteral nutrition, using larger numbers of well-matched patients, are required.

The traditional use of low residue diets in the management of patients with Crohn's disease has been questioned (Heaton *et al.* 1979). In an uncontrolled study this group reported that a high residue diet improved the clinical condition of their patients with Crohn's disease. Nevertheless, perhaps bowel rest may be of value during some periods in the treatment of inflammatory bowel disease, such as during an acute exacerbation, whereas a high residue diet may be preferable during remission.

SUMMARY

The role of bowel rest in the treatment of inflammatory bowel disease has yet to be ascertained. Its value in the treatment of ulcerative colitis seems doubtful but it may be useful in the treatment of Crohn's disease. Further controlled trials are required. However, the maintenance of a good state of nutrition by enteral or parenteral nutrition is likely to be of considerable benefit to patients suffering from these diseases.

REFERENCES

Brown JY (1913) The value of complete physiological rest of the large bowel in the treatment of certain ulcerative and obstructive lesions of this organ. *Surg. Gynecol Obstet*, **16**, 610–13.

Cattell RB (1948) The surgical treatment of ulcerative colitis. *Gastroenterology*, **10**, 63–66.

Dickinson RJ, Ashton MG, Axon ATR, Smith RC, Yeung CK & Hill GL (1980) Controlled trial of intravenous hyperalimentation and total bowel rest as an adjunct to the routine therapy of acute colitis. *Gastroenterology*, **79**, 1199–1204.

Dudrick SJ & Ruberg RL (1971) Principles and practice of parenteral nutrition. *Gastroenterology*, **61**, 901–910.

Dudrick SJ, MacFayden BV Jr & Daly JM (1976) Management of inflammatory bowel disease with parenteral hyperalimentation. In Clearfeld HR & Dinosos VP (eds). *Gastrointestinal Emergencies*, 193–199. Grune and Stratton, New York.

Harper PH, Truelove SC, Lee ECG, Kettlewell MGW, & Jewell DP (1983) Split ileostomy and ileocolostomy for Crohn's disease of the colon and ulcerative colitis: a 20 year survey. *Gut*, **24**, 106–13.

Heaton KW, Thornton JR & Emmett P (1979) Treatment of Crohn's disease with an unrefined carbohydrate, fibre-rich diet. *Br Med J*, **2**, 764–6.

Hill GL, Mair WSJ, Edwards JP & Goligher JC (1976) Decreased trypsin and bile acid in ileal fistula drainage during the administration of a chemically defined liquid elemental diet. *Br J Surg*, **63**, 133–6.

Homan WP & Kineen P (1978) Comparison of the results of resection bypass and bypass with exclusion for ileocaecal Crohn's disease. *Ann Surg*, **187**, 530–35.

Jones JH, Lennard-Jones JE & Lockhart-Mummery HE (1966) Experience in the treatment of Crohn's disease of the large intestine. *Gut*, **7**, 448–52.

Koudahl G. Kristensen M & Lenz K (1974) Bypass compared with resection for ileal Crohn's disease. *Scand J Gastroenterol*, **9**, 203–6.

Mullen JL, Hargrove WC, Dudrick SJ, Fitts WT & Rosato EF (1978) Ten years experience with intravenous hyperalimentation and inflammatory bowel disease. *Ann Surg*, **187**, 523–29.

Oberhelman HA, Kohatsu S, Taylor KB & Kivel RM (1968) Diverting Ileostomy in the surgical management of Crohn's disease of the colon. *Am J Surg*, **115**, 231–240.

O'Moràin C, Segal AW & Levi AJ (1984) Elemental diet as primary treatment of acute Crohn's disease: a controlled trial. *Br Med J*, **288**, 1859–62.

Reilly J, Ryan JA, Strole W & Fischer JE (1976) Hyperalimentation in inflammatory bowel disease. *Am J Surg*, **131**, 192–200.

Silk DBA (1974) Peptide absorption in man. *Gut*, **15** 494–501.

Truelove SC, Willoughby CP, Lee EG & Kettlewell MGW (1978) Further experience in the treatment of severe attacks of ulcerative colitis. *Lancet*, **ii**, 1086–88.

Weser E (1980) Total parenteral nutrition and bowel rest in inflammatory bowel disease. *Gastroenterology*, **79**, 1337.

Winitz M, Seedman DA & Graff J (1970) Studies in metabolic nutrition employing chemically defined diets. *Am J Clin Nutr*, **23**, 525–59.

Chapter 12 · Nutrition and Malignancy

The increasing availability of convenient and safe forms of enteral and parenteral nutrition has broadened the indications for their use. This has proved to be particularly valuable in the treatment of malignant diseases which have a profound effect on nutritional status. However, apart from direct mechanical causes, under-nutrition results from reduced oral intake, tumour host interactions and the effects of cancer therapy.

Reduced oral intake

Alterations in appetite

Loss of appetite in cancer patients is common. Taste abnormalities are frequently produced, and may make food unpalatable. The site of the tumour, type of treatment and psychological and emotional state of the patient are also known to play important roles. Even in the absence of a mechanical obstruction patients may experience a 'bloated feeling' after meals. This may be secondary to the central effects of malignancy but the atrophy of the gastrointestinal tract which occurs in cancer patients can be further exacerbated by a reduced oral intake, producing a vicious circle.

Direct effect on the gastrointestinal tract

Tumours often cause simple mechanical obstruction of the gastro-intestinal tract and this is most severe if sited proximally (oeso-phagus and stomach being notable clinical examples). More distal tumours generally produce less obvious but equally difficult problems, due to their insidious onset and frequent association with some degree of malabsorption.

Tumour host interactions

Complex hormonal and metabolic disturbances occur in patients
with malignant disease and several theories have been proposed to
explain the weight loss in patients with an adequate protein and
calorie intake. In 1948 Mider suggested that tumours may act as
'nitrogen traps' due to their more efficient use of amino acids
(Mider *et al.* 1948). However, much of this work was in small
animals and its application to the clinical situation has been
repeatedly questioned (Strain 1979).

It has been suggested for some time that by-products of tumour
cells may directly effect the metabolism of normal host cells, particularly gluconeogenesis, producing weight loss (Waterhouse
1974). This mechanism is thought to explain the observation that
increased lactic acid levels (due to anaerobic glycolysis and Cori
cycle activity) are only found in those cancer patients who exhibit
weight loss (Holroyde *et al.* 1975).

Weight loss resulting from cancer therapy

Adjuvent treatment for malignant disease, whether chemotherapy
or radiotherapy, is known to have a deleterious effect on nutritional status. Non-specific problems such as nausea, vomiting,
diarrhoea and malabsorption and specific problems particularly
glossitis, gastroenteritis and hepatobiliary disorders are well
recognized. The effects of radiotherapy are more often related to
the area being treated but with either form of treatment some
degree of malnutrition occurs in up to 80% of patients (Donaldson
1977). In addition chemotherapeutic agents may have direct
effects upon host tissues, possibly due to an inhibition of nucleic
acid synthesis (Stein *et al.* 1979).

Effects that have been described include:

Radiotherapy	*Chemotherapy*
nausea	nausea
vomiting and diarrhoea	vomiting and diarrhoea
radiation gastritis	oral ulceration

radiation enteritis
  chronic diarrhoea
  malabsorption

glossitis
mucosal changes
malabsorption
pancreatic dysfunction
diffuse hepatocellular
damage

NUTRITIONAL SUPPORT

Nutrition and tumour growth

Clearly it is essential to establish that improvements in nutrition do not result in rapid tumour development particularly with the demonstration in animals that improved calorie intake increased the tumour incidence (Tannenbaum & Silverstone 1953). It has been alleged that reversing a nutritional defect will alter the host immune response and indeed, forced feeding has been shown to be deleterious in the absence of adjuvent therapy (Terepka & Waterhouse 1956). However, the converse seems to apply in small animals given normal rather than supranormal nutrition where it has been possible to demonstrate an improved tumour response rate (Daly *et al.* 1980). Clinical studies support this (Copeland *et al.* 1977). Although with this latter effect it is important to differentiate between an improved response rate and improvements due to an increased tolerance to adjuvent therapy, it seems that nutritional support improves tumour response rates and reduces toxic side-effects. Furthermore, there is no direct evidence that 'feeding the patient, feeds the tumour'.

Nutrition and the patient

Nutritional defects due to inadequate intake can usually be rapidly reversed simply by refeeding and in this respect enteral nutrition is always preferable. In some patients, however, simple refeeding fails to establish a significant degree of anabolism and animal work supports the clinical observation that an adequate intake does not always preserve lean body mass (LBM). Moreover it has been shown that forced feeding in this situation often simply results in an increased nitrogen excretion. Patients and animals with malignancies it seems do not handle exogenous nitrogen and calories in the same fashion as normal individuals (Fischer 1984).

Whilst simple refeeding often fails to preserve LBM there is some evidence for experimental animals that this loss is not obligatory, but supplementary measures, such as exercise, insulin and branched chain amino acids are probably required to manipulate the host metabolism (Moley *et al*. 1984).

Patient assessment and monitoring

This is covered in detail elsewhere in this book.

Indications and methods of feeding

Enteral nutrition should always be instituted (or reinstituted) where possible but initially it may be necessary to control side-effects of adjuvent therapy such as nausea, vomiting and diarrhoea. If these are prolonged, parenteral nutrition can be employed as a temporary measure and is often rewarded by a rapid clinical improvement and a surprising return of appetite. Other problems limiting oral intake such as alterations in taste and anorexia have no specific remedies and can only be managed by a careful and persuasive approach by a dietitian (see p. 74). Some discipline may be required to ensure that the nutritional therapy is being taken.

Where local oral problems are troublesome and cannot be managed by simple oral hygiene and the elimination of fungal infections, a fine bore feeding tube may be necessary. These can be used to advantage intermittently and/or on an outpatient basis.

Although parenteral nutrition for cancer patients remains controversial its use is expanding in three main areas:

1 **Pre-treatment therapy:** To improve the nutritional status of malnourished patients prior to surgery or adjuvent cancer therapy
2 **Peri-treatment:** To decrease or limit the morbidity and mortality associated with curative surgery and aggressive chemotherapeutic regimes

3 **Post-treatment:** Nutritional support can be continued into the convalescent period when oral intake remains inadequate. This also includes those patients who, due to surgical resections (production of the short bowel syndrome) or continuing malignant disease (where surgical treatment is not possible or there is recurrent disease) need supplementary nutritional support, including home parenteral nutrition (HTPN).

In all treatment groups the aim is to improve the nutritional status of the host but not the tumour.

When parenteral therapy is unavoidable, standard regimes are advisable as there is general agreement that supranormal calories and nitrogen are of no advantage and probably harmful to the host. Patients must be chosen with care, and although some authorities include terminal malignancy as an indication for long-term and HTPN, psychological and social factors must be considered prior to this major undertaking.

REFERENCES

Copeland EM, Daly JM & Dudrick SJ (1977) Nutrition as an adjunct to cancer treatment. *Cancer Res*, **37**, 2451–2456.

Daly JJ, Reynolds HM, Rowlands BJ, Dudrick SJ & Copeland EM (1980) Nutritional manipulation and chemotherapeutic response in the rat. *Ann Surg*, **190**, 316–322.

Donaldson SS (1977) Nutritional consequences of radiotherapy. *Cancer Res*, **37**, 2407–2413.

Fischer JE (1984) Adjuvant parenteral nutrition in the patient with cancer. *Surgery*, **96**, 578–580.

Holroyde CP, Gabuzda TG, Dutnam RC *et al.* (1975) Altered glucose metabolism in metastatic carcinoma. *Cancer Res*, **35** 3710–3714.

Mider GB, Tesluk H & Morton JJ (1948) Effects of Walker carcinoma 256 on food intake, body weight and nitrogen metabolism of growing rats. *Acta Un Int Cancer*, **6**, 409–420.

Moley JF, Morrison S & Norton JA (1983) Effects of exogenous insulin administration on food intake, body weight change and tumour doubling time. *Surg Forum*, **34**, 91–3.

Stein TP, Hargrave WC, Miller EE *et al.* (1979) Effect of nutritional status and 5-Fluorouracil on protein synthesis in parenterally alimented Lew/Mai rats. *J Nat Cancer Inst*, **63**, 379–382.

Strain AJ (1979) Cancer cachexia in man: a review. *Invest Cell Pathol*, **2**, 181–193.

Tannenbaum A & Silverstone H (1953) Nutrition in relation to cancer. *Adv Cancer Res* (New York: Academic Press), **1**, 451–56.

Terepka AR & Waterhouse C (1956) Metabolic observations during the forced feeding of patients with cancer. *Am J Med*, **20**, 225–238.

Waterhouse C (1974) How tumours effect host metabolism. *Ann NY Acad Sci*, **230**, 86–93.

Chapter 13 · Nutrition in Renal Failure

INTRODUCTION

Renal failure produces a number of metabolic and fluid balance problems which make the administration of enteral and parenteral nutrition more difficult than usual (see Table 13.1). Before dialysis was available patients with renal failure were managed by fluid, electrolyte and protein restriction and a high intake of non-protein calories. Such restrictions were incompatible with adequate nutritional support. With the availability of dialysis, management was made easier but there remained the problem of limiting fluid volume in oligo/anuric patients. Excess fluid volume had to be

Table 13.1. Additional problems in the administration of nutritional support to patients with renal failure.

Fluid balance
The volume of fluid administered is limited to the volume of urine and other output or the amount of fluid removed by dialysis or haemofiltration

Metabolic
Failure to excrete protein breakdown products
Metabolic acidosis
Insulin 'resistance'
Possible delayed lipid clearance
Hyperkalaemia
Hypocalcaemia + hyperphosphataemia
A hypermetabolic state is common especially in multiple trauma, infections, and corticosteroid treatment
Liver failure may also be present

Clinical
Susceptibility to infection increased
Anaemia common

Practical
Access to the circulation is required for both dialysis and parenteral nutrition
Protein and amino acid losses are exacerbated by peritoneal dialysis
Amino acids are lost on dialysis

removed at a daily 3–4 hour haemodialysis session or by continuous peritoneal dialysis. This problem has been overcome by
the development of continuous arterio-venous haemofiltration,
which allows virtually unrestricted volumes of fluid and full nutritional support to be administered. Whether this advance will
reduce the persisting high mortality in ARF remains to be established, but it is likely that patients who are well dialysed, adequately nourished and in fluid balance will fare better than before.

ACUTE RENAL FAILURE (ARF)

ARF commonly presents as a complication of a serious underlying
illness, trauma or surgery. The patients are therefore often in a
hypermetabolic state with an increased breakdown of protein
leading to the release of urea, potassium and hydrogen ions which
they are unable to excrete. Moreover, the patients are often
reluctant or unable to take a normal diet by mouth. Even in established reversible ARF one has to face a period of 2–3 weeks during
which the patient is too ill to consume an adequate diet. The
provision of sufficient calories reduces endogenous protein breakdown and urea production so it is imperative that nutritional
support be planned early rather than late. There is, however, no
evidence that nutritional support hastens recovery from ARF.

When the presence of established renal failure has been confirmed arrangements for dialysis should be made immediately.
There is no advantage in delaying dialysis until hyperkalaemia or
uraemia complications make it mandatory. Dialysis should be
started when the plasma urea is > 30 mmol/1 or the potassium is
> 6 mmol/1 or if fluid removal is required. The kind of dialysis
and nutritional support for each patient must be planned to suit
individual circumstances and the following scheme provides basic
guidelines.

In the presence of decreased renal excretion, the rate of the rise
in blood urea can be used to assess the rate of protein breakdown
(Table 13.2 and p. 104). The rate of protein breakdown will dictate
the frequency of dialysis and the quantities of protein or amino
acids to be administered.

Table 13.2.

Category	Rise in blood urea	Protein breakdown
	(mmol/l/day)	g nitrogen/day
Mild	4–8	5–10
Intermediate	8–12	10–15
Hypermetabolic	12	15

Can the patient be managed without dialysis?

Patients with some residual renal function (creatinine clearance > 10 ml/min) can be managed without dialysis provided that they are not hypermetabolic. In adults the volume of fluid intake per day is restricted to 500 ml plus the previous 24 hour urinary output. Additional allowances must be made for fluid losses from burns, nasogastric aspiration, fistulae, diarrhoea or excessive sweating. Protein should be restricted to 0.5 g of protein/kg body weight/day (80 mg nitrogen/kg/day) and 40 kcals/kg/day of energy must be provided. The daily electrolyte requirement should be calculated from losses rather than applying blanket restriction on potassium and sodium intake. Usual requirements are 40 mmol of Na^+ and K^+/day. Patients with polyuric renal failure (e.g. following acute tubular necrosis or relief of urinary obstruction) may require sodium and potassium supplements rather than restriction.

Dialysis—peritoneal or haemo? (Table 13.3)

Peritoneal dialysis is very useful in the management of uraemic emergencies because it is simple to perform, universally available and corrects metabolic derangements gradually. It is particularly useful when the clinical situation is less severe and a short period of dialysis is all that is required. It is not troublefree and there can be problems with catheter insertion, dialysate flow, peritonitis and hyperglycaemia. Both protein and amino-acids are lost during peritoneal dialysis (see Table 13.3).

For the hypermetabolic patient a combination of haemodialysis

Table 13.3. Comparison of haemo—and peritoneal dialysis

Haemodialysis + haemofiltration

Advantages	Disadvantages
Best in the hypermetabolic patient	Requires specialized equipment and staff
	Vascular access
	Amino acid losses = 1.5 – 3.0 g/hour
	Anticoagulation required
	Hypotension

Peritoneal dialysis

Advantages	Disadvantages
Universally available	Complications of catheter insertion
Useful in: hypotensive patients	Peritonitis
: bleeding patients	Protein losses (0.5 g/litre)
Dialysis glucose available as calories source	Amino acid losses (0.35 g/litre)
Easy fluid removal	Not recommended after abdominal surgery
Gradual correction of metabolic derangements	

and continuous haemofiltration is the best method. Technically this is more complicated, requiring specialized equipment and staff and reliable vascular access.

The vascular access for haemofiltration and dialysis can be via femoral and arterial lines but a double lumen central venous catheter or Scribner shunt is preferable. The haemofilter is set to produce 6 litres of filtrate/day which provides a creatinine clearance of approximately 4 ml/min in the average adult. The haemofiltration is continuous, interrupted only by haemodialysis treatment, the frequency of which can be reduced and need not include fluid removal. A typical regimen is shown in Table 13.4.

What are the calorie, protein, vitamin, mineral and fluid requirements?

The calorie and nitrogen requirements will depend on the meta-

Table 13.4. Typical fluid and parenteral nutrition regimen for patient on haemofiltration (6 litres/day)

Vol.		K Calories	Sodium
1.0 litres	Vamin 9-glucose	400	50 mmol
1.5 litres	20% Dextrose	1200	–
0.5 litres	20% Intralipid	1000	–
1.0 litres	1.8% Sodium chloride	–	300 mmol
2.0 litres	0.9% Sodium chloride	–	300 mmol
0.5 litres	8.4% Sodium bicarbonate	–	150 mmol
—			
6.5 litres		2600	800 mmol

bolic state (see p. 11). Water-soluble vitamins are removed by dialysis but the standard daily doses more than compensate for these losses. There is usually no reason to try to normalize the plasma calcium and phosphate for they will stabilize at acceptable levels with adequate dialysis and the administration of phosphate binders. Special care is needed however in patients with rhabdomyolysis and the tumour lysis syndrome when changes in calcium and phosphate levels are particularly marked. Phosphate in parenteral nutrition solutions should be restricted initially but supplements are needed if haemofiltration is used, and during the recovery phase. Supplementation of magnesium and zinc may be required because, although their renal excretion is reduced, loss can occur by other routes e.g. fistulae, and the nutritional stimulus to tissue repair will increase the requirements. Sodium and potassium requirements can be calculated on an individual basis depending on losses. Dialysis and haemofiltration allow flexibility in calculating the sodium and potassium allowances but excessive sodium and potassium administration between haemodialysis can lead to problems, especially in hypermetabolic patients.

Fluid intake has also to be calculated on an individual basis and although imbalances can be corrected by dialysis, rapid removal of fluid can cause troublesome hypotension. The volume of fluid administered is determined by what can be safely tolerated by the patient (i.e. avoiding fluid overload) and what can be comfortably removed by dialysis or ultrafiltration. Continuous haemofiltration solves the problem by maintaining the patient in continuous fluid balance.

By what route should the nutritional support be administered?

If the gastrointestinal tract is available but the patient is unable to take a full diet by mouth, then tube feeding should be considered. If the patient is on continuous peritoneal dialysis, rigid sodium, potassium and fluid restriction is not required. The feed can therefore be constituted on standard lines. Any positive fluid balance can be dialysed off using a more concentrated dialysis solution for some of the cycles.

If the patient is being intermittently haemodialysed the volume of enteral feed should be restricted to 2.5 litres/day and sodium and potassium intake will have to be limited to 60 mmol/day each. With haemofiltration there is no fluid restriction.

Parenteral nutrition is reserved for the patients in whom the gastrointestinal tract is unavailable. A central venous catheter rather than peripheral veins should be used because if these thrombose they will not be available as future blood access sites should the patient eventually require chronic maintenance haemodialysis.

There are a number of amino acid solutions available, some are constituted without electrolytes and these are useful because they allow one to add precisely the quantities of sodium, potassium and phosphate required. A potential problem with the use of synthetic amino acid solutions is the production of a metabolic acidosis (p. 118).

Lipid emulsion does not interfere with dialysis and can be used in renal failure.

Insulin supplements are often required because of the insulin resistance encountered in hypermetabolic renal failure patients. It is best administered intravenously by continuous infusion (p. 105). The dose is adjusted according to a sliding scale based on hourly capillary blood sample measurements until the needs are known.

Insulin requirements can be large (200–300 units/day). All peritoneal dialysis fluids contain glucose and this can be used by the patient as a calorie source but insulin may be required.

Amino acids are removed by haemodialysis at the rate of 1.5–3.0 g/hour (i.e. 0.2–0.5 g N/hour) and this must be allowed for in the daily nitrogen prescription.

It is necessary to monitor the following:

1　Daily plasma urea, creatinine, electrolytes. Glucose should be checked at least six hourly but more frequent capillary blood samples are initially required to adjust insulin doses. pH and base deficit should be checked daily initially to see whether the institution of i.v. feeding is causing or aggravating the metabolic acidosis.

2　Measurement of urinary electrolyte losses allows one to calculate the minimum sodium and potassium that can be administered.

3　At first daily, then twice weekly calcium, phosphate and albumin.

4　When practical daily weighing gives a guide to fluid balance.

Chronic renal failure

The management of the long-term maintenance haemodialysis patient who requires nutritional support (e.g. after major gastrointestinal surgery) is no different from that of patients in acute renal failure. For those patients not yet established on dialysis the problem is less pressing, for some adaptation to the reduction in renal function is present but temporary dialysis support maybe needed.

Renal transplantation

The only additional factor in these patients is that they are usually receiving high doses of corticosteroids which increase susceptibility to infection, produce insulin resistance and aggravate the negative nitrogen balance.

Table 13.5. Nutritional support in renal failure

Is dialysis required?		
No	**Yes**	
if	if	
(a) Residual creatinine clearance > 10 ml/min	(a) Residual creatinine clearance < 10 ml/min	
(b) The patient is not hypermetabolic	(b) The patient is hypermetabolic	
	(c) Acute metabolic or fluid overload problems	
Fluids = 500 ml/day + losses		
Protein = 0.5 g/kg/day		
Energy = 40 kcal/kg/day	Peritoneal	Haemodialysis/filtration

Can full diet be consumed?

No

Gastro intestinal tract available

Yes   No

Enteral nutrition   Parenteral nutrition

Summary (Table 13.5)

Renal failure patients are a potentially difficult group for whom to provide nutritional support. It should be started as soon as possible using the enteral route whenever possible, and the parenteral route when it is not. Fluid and electrolyte balance is more difficult than in the patients with normal renal function but the combination of dialysis and haemofiltration has simplified management.

FURTHER READING

Abel RN, Beck CH (Jr), Abbott M, Ryan JA (Jr), Barrett GO & Fish JE (1973) Improved survival from acute renal failure after treatment with intravenous L-amino acids and glucose. *New Engl J Med*, **288**, 695-99.

Dodd NJ, O'Donovan RM, Bennett-Jones DN, Rylance PB, Bewick M, Parsons V & Weston MJ (1983) Arteriovenous haemofiltration: a recent advance in the management of renal failure. *Br Med J*, **287**, 1008-10.

Goldstein MB (1983) Acute Renal Failure. in: *Medical Clinics of North America*, **67**, 1325-41.

Kjellestrand CM, Pru CE, Jahnke WR & Davin TD (1983) *Acute renal failure in Replacement of Renal Function by Dialysis* 536-68. 2nd Edition eds W Drukker, FM Parsons and JF Maher Martinus Nijoff, Boston.

Wesson DE, Mitch WE & Wilmore DE (1983) Nutritional considerations in the treatment of acute renal failure. Chapter 24, *Acute Renal Failure* eds. BM Brenner and JM Lazarus WB Saunders Co, Philadelphia.

Chapter 14 · Nutrition in Liver Disease

INTRODUCTION

Patients with liver disease are commonly malnourished. A survey in the UK demonstrated that between 40–50% of patients, hospitalized for chronic liver disease, had significant reductions in the various nutritional parameters (O'Keefe *et al.* 1980). The explanation is complex, but includes the anorexia that usually accompanies any form of ill-health, alcohol abuse, drug side-effects, and excessive protein restriction in patients with porto-systemic encephalopathy. It is the latter condition that is most responsible for the fear clinicians have in recommending a normal diet to their patients with liver disease. Furthermore, the clinician is often misled by the fact that significant weight loss may be masked by fluid retention and oedema in the cirrhotic patient. Significant depletion of body stores, in particular protein, is associated with reduced host-defence. Patients with liver disease are particularly at risk from spontaneous infections as a consequence of a wide variety of defects in immunocompetence (McKay 1975). Whilst only some of these defects have been related to malnutrition, these are potentially reversible with the appropriate nutritional support.

The most controversial area of nutrition in liver disease relates to protein.

In chronic liver disease numerous studies have shown that patients with cirrhosis and portal hypertension become 'intolerant' of protein as demonstrated by the reduced ability to metabolize excess dietary intake. The defect particularly affects aromatic amino acid and ammonia clearance since both are metabolized and excreted via the liver. Only the branched chain amino acids can be oxidized outside the liver. The resultant accumulation of ammonia and aromatic amino acids within the plasma is toxic resulting in neurological disturbance, commonly termed 'hepatic encephalopathy'. It may therefore seem appropriate to exclude protein from the diet. Such measures, taken together with bowel purgation and sterilization, have traditionally formed the backbone of medical management of liver failure. However, the approach ignores the basic maintenance requirements to cover losses due to the 'wear and tear' of endogenous protein turnover. Furthermore, whilst protein oxidation rates are suppressed, they continue, albeit at lower levels than normal, resulting in inevitable protein depletion. Although few studies of protein requirements have been made, a study of ours indicated that at least 40 g first class protein should be given (O'Keefe *et al.* 1981b). If the diet was given by slow constant infusion, even greater quantities could be given (i.e. 70–80 g/d)* without any demonstrable effect on encephalopathy or accumulation of amino acids in the plasma (O'Keefe *et al.* 1981a). In addition, these studies demonstrated that whole body turnover rates were over twice normal in patients with fulminant hepatic failure, with less major increases in patients with cirrhosis. We therefore concluded that the protein should be given together with high intakes of glucose in order to suppress protein catabolism. Such regimens would be strongly anabolic, and, via the induced insulin response, may well potentiate hepatic regeneration (Farivar *et al.* 1976).

Nutritional support for patients with acute liver disease can be equally important, but for different reasons. In this instance, the problem is one of metabolic homeostasis rather than nutritional deficiency. Besides preventing amino acid accumulation, the liver also complements the actions of the endocrine pancreas in maintaining a remarkably constant blood glucose concentration during periods of starvation or negative energy balance. Patients developing fulminant hepatic failure commonly become comatosed, with irreversible brain damage, due to hypoglycaemia. Under these conditions the provision of a constant infusion of glucose can be life-saving, buying enough time to allow for the remarkable capacity of the liver to regenerate. Liver biopsies taken

---

*6.25 g protein or 'amino acids' = 1 g nitrogen.

from fatal cases often have histological evidence of active regeneration. Since these patients often are hypermetabolic, concentrated glucose infusion will offer further benefits of decreasing catabolism and increasing anabolism as outlined in the previous paragraph.

The main nutritional deficiencies referred to above involve protein and energy. However, deficiency of micronutrients are possible also. Demonstration of an improvement in prothrombin time after parenteral—as opposed to enteral—therapy, is strongly suggestive of Vitamin K deficiency. The deficiency is more common in patients with biliary stasis, since bile is a co-factor in the absorption of the fat soluble Vitamins A, D, K and E. It therefore follows that malabsorption of the remaining vitamins, and dietary fat, should co-exist. Some evidence has been obtained showing patients with chronic biliary disease to have 'hepatic osteodystrophy' which is partly responsive to parenteral Vitamin D, and oral calcium administration (Skinner *et al.* 1977). These observations lend support to the practice of providing patients surffering from prolonged biliary stasis with monthly injections of the fat soluble vitamins. Requirements of water soluble vitamins, have also been shown to be elevated in patients with chronic liver disease. Decreased plasma and tissue concentrations have been associated with not only decreased intake, but also increased urinary losses (McIntyre 1979).

CLASSIFICATION

Liver diseases can be classified according to their different nutritional requirements. Each category is considered in turn.

Chronic liver diseases

    Cirrhosis
        a   Uncomplicated
        b   Hypoalbuminaemia and fluid retention
        c   Encephalopathy
    Alcoholic
    Biliary tract

Acute liver diseases

Viral and drug hepatitis
Alcoholic
Fulminant hepatic failure
Biliary tract

Chronic liver disease

Uncomplicated cirrhosis

All aetiologies included. A normal balanced diet should be encouraged. It should contain at least 60–80 g first-class protein together with between 2000–3000 kcal/d depending upon the level of physical activity. A high carbohydrate, low fat diet is often more acceptable, especially in patients with pancreatic or biliary tract involvement, but should never be enforced. Multivitamin and bran supplementation may be given as required.

Weight changes are difficult to assess due to fluid retention problems, and attention must be given to a good dietary history. Other physical parameters of the assessment of nutritional status such as clinical evidence of muscle-wasting, triceps skinfold thicknesses or midarm circumferences, are also useful in the follow-up of the individual patient provided an experienced person is responsible for these measurements.

Cirrhosis, with hypoalbuminaemia, ascites and peripheral oedema: non-encephalopathic

The mechanism of fluid retention in cirrhosis is complex. However, plasma oncotic pressure is commonly low due to reduced albumin concentrations. Sodium concentrations are also often misleadingly low due to a dilution effect: total body sodium is in fact elevated as a consequence of increased aldosterone activity. Thus treatment should include salt and fluid restriction (20–40 mmol sodium/day, 1000–1500 ml fluid), anti-aldosterone drugs (e.g. spironolactone) and dietary protein should be increased to 80–120 g/day. The practical problem that ensues is that dietary protein contains a lot of salt, and severe salt restriction in cooking results in tasteless food.

However, such measures are often only temporary until fluid retention is reversed (c.g. 2–3 weeks), whereupon salt intake may be increased with the advice 'no added salt'. In so-called 'resistant ascites' patients, natriuretic drugs may have to be used in order to increase dietary allowances. Sudden decompression of ascitic fluid by tapping must be avoided unless the intra-abdominal pressure becomes so great that it interferes with normal respiration. This procedure can not only precipitate renal failure but also results in further loss of body proteins.

Cirrhosis with encephalopathy

As stated in the introduction, encephalopathy has been associated with a disturbance in protein metabolism and protein intolerance. However, there is no single aetiology to encephalopathy. Numerous other associations include electrolyte imbalance, bacterial or drug toxaemia, hypoglycaemia, and disturbed fat metabolism. Therefore, it should be proven that protein intolerance is the cause before protein restriction is used in further management. This can be done by initially screening the blood for electrolyte, glucose and bacteriological abnormalities and then reducing protein intake to 40 g/day. This level must not be reduced as negative nitrogen balance will occur. Such intakes, given in three equal portions during the day will not induce or worsen encephalopathy. On improvement of encephalopathy, protein intake should be increased in stepwise increments of 20 g every three days until, either intake reaches 80 g/day or encephalopathy returns. Should the latter occur, reasonable evidence is obtained that the patient is protein intolerant. In addition, information on 'tolerance level' is gained. As outlined in the introduction, the protein must be given together with a high intake of carbohydrate (e.g. 'Polycal') in an attempt to suppress endogenous protein breakdown. The importance of this lies in the observation that the contribution by catabolism to the amino acid load on the liver is 4–6 times greater than that of the normal dietary intake (O'Keefe *et al.* 1981b).

Branched chain amino acids

Much recent evidence has accumulated to support the usefulness of these amino acids in the treatment of hepatic encephalopathy. From a theoretical viewpoint they should be well-tolerated in patients with liver failure since they are oxidized extrahepatically in muscle. In this way the nitrogen intake can be increased. In a recent multi-centre controlled trial in America, Horst *et al.* (1984) compared two groups of protein intolerant cirrhotic patients. They were fed either standard or branched chain enriched amino acid solution until they attained an intake of 80 g of protein per day or the equivalent, or until they developed stage II encephalopathy. Seven of the twenty patients from the standard protein group and only one out of seventeen in the branched chain enriched group developed encephalopathy. Furthermore, plasma amino acid profiles showed an increase in branched chain amino acids in the study group and thus they were able to conclude that oral branched chain amino acid supplements appeared to induce positive nitrogen balance to approximately the same degree as an equivalent amount of dietary protein without inducing encephalopathy as frequently. Fischer and Baldassarini (1976), suggested that the improvement in encephalopathy was a result of the improvement in plasma amino acid profiles which indirectly reduced the uptake of aromatic amino acids into the brain and thus reduced false neurotransmitter synthesis. We (O'Keefe *et al.* 1981a) also demonstrated that branched amino acids are anti-catabolic and may therefore reduce the catabolic state associated with liver failure (1981b). However, once encephalopathy has been reversed, supplements are probably unnecessary and certainly not cost-effective. They are presently available in either oral (e.g. Hepatamine, Scientific Hospital Supplies, or Hepatonutril, Oxford Nutrition) or intravenous form (4% solution, Travenol Laboratories) with a recommended supplementation of about 40 g/day.

NB. It must be stressed that branched chain amino acids should not be given alone for any length of time as the mixture is incomplete and therefore cannot maintain protein synthesis without further addition of the other essential amino acids.

Chronic alcoholic liver disease

In the early stages the liver is not cirrhotic, but abnormally loaded with fat. This may be associated with a mild hepatitis picture. Nutritional regimens for these individuals are the same as for those with uncomplicated cirrhosis. However, the recommendation of a balanced diet is often ignored, since the consumption of alcohol often dominates their lives. Consequently, relative deficiencies of protein, vitamins and trace elements (e.g. zinc and magnesium) are extremely common in chronic alcoholics. With the progression to cirrhosis these deficiencies are exacerbated. Water soluble vitamin deficiencies often complicate the disease and may manifest themselves as dermatoses or mental abnormalities, e.g. Wernicke-Korsakoff Syndrome. In such patients it is incorrect to wait for the symptoms to subside before instituting a normal diet. In the absence of severe diarrhoea, nasogastric feeding should be commenced with one of the available liquid formula diets (see pp. 240–44). Whilst oral multi-vitamin supplements are sufficient in most patients, those with neurological disturbance should be given daily parenteral injections. Psychiatric rehabilitation is an essential part of treatment and should include advice on replacing excessive alcohol intakes with three nourishing meals a day.

Chronic biliary tract disease

The important difference in this group of patients with regard to diet is that fat and fat soluble vitamin absorption will decrease with increasing biliary stasis. Bile salts act as detergents within the gut lumen, breaking down dietary fat into an absorbable form ('micelles'). Therefore it is wise to avoid large intakes of dietary fat particularly if the symptoms of steatorrhoea occur (i.e. abdominal distension, diarrhoea, excessive flatus, foul-smelling pale stoods). In these patients dietary fat should be replaced wherever possible with medium chain triglycerides which are not subject to the micellar digestion/absorption system (see p. 81). In addition montly parenteral injections of fat soluble vitamins (i.e. Vitamins A, D, K and E) should be given. Such treatment should correct calcium malabsorption. However, although hypocalcaemia is rare, it is customary to continue to supply dietary calcium supplements (e.g. effervescent calcium).

Decrease in absorption can also occur without clinical evidence of steatorrhoea and therefore should always be assessed by measuring the response of the prothrombin time to parenteral injection of Vitamin K. This group of patients may manage on increased oral supplements. Again, a trial should be undertaken to ascertain this possibility. Plasma calcium, magnesium, phosphate, and bone-specific alkaline phosphatase should be checked in order to detect overt abnormalities in Vitamin D metabolism.

Acute liver disease

Acute hepatitis (due to virus and drugs)

The disease is characterized by an acute illness associated with jaundice and raised liver enzymes (e.g. aspartate transaminase). Most attacks are transient, a small proportion progressing, either rapidly to fulminant hepatic failure (see below), or slowly to chronic liver disease (see above). Requirements for protein and energy are essentially the same as those for a moderately hypermetabolic illness, with increased requirements of protein to about 120 g/day. Energy requirement is approximately 2000 kcal/day and is generally given in the form of glucose, although recent studies have shown that dietary fat or soya-bean oil emulsions (e.g. Intralipid) may be given to provide 50% of total caloric intake. The fear of giving lipid to patients with liver disease, is probably based on early experience with lipid emulsions where sensitivities to certain components occurred. However, there have been no recent reports for any such problems with intravenous fat provided it is given as described above. Active intervention along these lines has been shown to be effective in reducing the duration of illness (Chalmers *et al.* 1955).

Hypoglycaemia and encephalopathy rarely occur and when noted may indicate serious progression to fulminant hepatic failure. Vitamin supplementation is advised since hepatic necrosis will be associated with increased loss of hepatic stores via urinary excretion.

Acute alcoholic hepatitis

Treatment should be along the lines suggested above. However, since these patients usually have a long history of alcohol abuse and the associated neglect of dietary intake, nutritional support should be commenced immediately on admission to hospital. A recent, controlled study has shown that supplementation of the ad-lib ward diet (estimated at about 100 g protein plus 3000 kcal/day) with 70–85 g of intravenous amino acids daily, resulted in increased survival and plasma biochemical improvement (Nasrallah & Calambos 1980). These results are encouraging for the reason that although most patients only develop mild hepatitis which responds to alcohol withdrawal, a small section progress insidiously to irreversible liver damage, sub-acute hepatic necrosis and death. Nutritional support in the latter group should follow that outlined below for fulminant hepatic failure.

Fulminant hepatic failure

For reasons presently unknown, some patients with hepatitis progress to this disease characterized by massive hepatic necrosis (indicated by AST 1000 u/l and prothrombin time 30 seconds— Vitamin K un-responsive) and mortality rates between 70–80%. The conscious state deteriorates rapidly. The duration of the illness is short, the patient either dying within a week in a comatosed state, or recovering completely. In the latter group, the regenerative capacity of the liver is so spectacular that histology taken six months later can be totally normal.

Nutrition has two equally important roles in the acute medical management of fulminant hepatic failure. Firstly, it can provide 'hepatic support' by taking over the gluconeogenic functions of the liver, thereby ensuring a constant supply of glucose vital for nervous tissue respiration. In normal man, hepatic glucose output has been estimated to be 180 g/day (Cahill 1970). Secondly it can suppress protein catabolism, increase anabolism, and therefore optimize conditions for hepatic regeneration. We have shown that the intravenous infusion of amino acid/glucose solutions to provide 3 g amino acids/hour and 5 g/hour glucose is well tolerated, resulting in decreased catabolism, improved plasma amino acid profiles and increased insulin concentrations. Although the usefulness of branched chain enriched solutions in this situation is unclear, it seems logical to use a branched chain enriched mixture rather than the standard preparation if it is available. Insulin is thought to be the key hormone influencing hepatic regeneration (Farivar *et al.* 1976), probably through its strong anabolic potential.

Oral intake should be discontinued because of the risks of ileus and inhalation. Parenteral feeding should be instituted along the lines suggested above. Close attention has to be paid to central venous pressure and renal output as coincident renal failure is common.

Acute biliary tract disease

This group of patients are characterized by colicky right upper quadrant abdominal pain, nausea and vomiting. Early stages may not be associated with jaundice but with progression plasma bilirubin and alkaline phosphatase rise rapidly, resulting in icterus, dark urine and pale stools. Initial management includes fluid and electrolyte replacement, investigation of the site of obstruction, and finally surgical intervention. If the block is successfully cleared, further care is as for a postoperative patient.

If unsuccessful, fat and fat soluble vitamin malabsorption might result necessitating the use of dietary MCT rather than LCT and intravenous vitamin supplementation. When a long-term biliary drainage tube is left *in situ*, it is sometimes helpful to reinfuse the bile into the stomach, although in practice this is difficult. Alternatively, tube feeding with a diet which does not require digestion such as an elemental preparation (eg MCT Pepdite 2 + or Peptisorbon see p. 244) can be used until such time as the normal anatomy and physiology of the gastrointestinal tract is reinstituted.

TPN hepatitis

The majority of patients on long-term TPN develop mild, but usually reversible, changes in liver function tests, e.g. elevation of alkaline phosphatase and gamma-glutaryl transferase enzymes (O'Keefe *et al.* 1985). In severe cases this can evolve into frank cholestasis. The most common cause is excessive intravenous caloric intakes, but chronic sepsis, endotoxaemia and biliary sludge formation have also been invoked in aetiology. Measures should include a reduction in total caloric intake with an increase in fat calories to provide between 30 and 40% of total caloric intake. Chronic sepsis should be investigated with the appropriate ultrasound or CT scan investigations.

REFERENCES

Cahill GF (1970) starvation in man. *N Engl J Med*, **291**, 668–75.

Chalmers TC, Eckhardt RD, Reynolds WE *et al.* (1955) The treatment of acute infective hepatitis; studies of the effects of diet, rest, physical reconditioning on the acute course of the disease and on the incidence of relapse and residual abnormalities. *J Clin Invest*, **34**, 1163–1235.

Farivar M, Bucher NLR, Wands J *et al.* (1976) Beneficial effects of *insulin* and glucagon on fulminant murine hepatitis. *Gastroenterology*, **70**, 981.

Fischer JE & Baldassarini RJ (1976) Pathogenesis and therapy of hepatic coma. Popper H & Schaffner F (eds) *Progress in Liver Diseases*, **V**, 363–697. Grune & Stratton, New York.

Horst D, Grace ND, Conn HO *et al.* (1984) Comparison of dietary protein with an oral branched enriched amino acid supplement in chronic portal systemic encephalopathy analysed controlled trial. *Hepatology*, **IV**, No. 2 279–87.

McIntyre N & Morgan MY (1979) Wright R ed. *Liver and Biliary Disease*. 114–116. WB Saunders Co Ltd, London.

McKay IR (1975) Immunologic disorders in liver disease. Schiff L ed. *Diseases of the Liver*, 4th edn. JB Lippincott Co, Philadelphia.

Nasrallah SM & Galambos JT (1980) Amino acid therapy of alcoholic hepatitis. *Lancet*, **ii**, 1276–7.

O'Keefe SJ, Bean E, Symmonds K *et al.* (1985) Clinical evaluation of the '3-in1' intravenous nutrient solution. *SA Med J*, **68**, 82–6.

O'Keefe SJ, Abraham RR, Davis M & Williams R (1981a) Protein turnover in acute and chronic liver disease. Wright PD ed. 2nd European Congress on Parenteral and Enteral Nutrition, *Acta Chirur Scand, Suppl*, **507**, 91–101.

O'Keefe SJ, El-Zayadi AR, Carraher TE, Davis M & Williams R (1980) Malnutrition and immunoincompetence in patients with liver disease. *Lancet*, **ii**, 615–17.

O'Keefe SJ, Abraham RR, El-Zayadi AR, Davis M & Williams R (1981b) Increased plasma tyrosine concentrations in patients with cirrhosis and fulminant hepatic failure associated with increased plasma flux and reduced hepatic oxidation capacity. *Gastroenterology*, **81**, 1017–24.

Skinner RK, Long RG, Sherlock S *et al.* (1977) 25-hydroxylation of Vitamin D in primary biliary cirrhosis. *Lancet*, **i**, 720–21.

Chapter 15 · Nutrition in Sepsis

The metabolic changes associated with sepsis are complex, imperfectly understood and controversial. It is only recently that systems to grade the severity of sepsis have emerged (Elubate & Stoner 1983; Stevens 1983); it is to be hoped that the refinement of such scoring schemes will promote a clearer understanding of the metabolic perturbations and thus enable treatment to be applied with greater precision.

The acute-phase response to infection includes an augmentation of neutrophils and lymphocytes. Several leukocyte products initiate a spectrum of inflammatory responses including the more widespread effects of the peptide interleukin one on the secretion of hepatocyte acute phase proteins, on aspects of the repair process and on amplification of muscle proteolysis. Septic endotoxins also have metabolic consequence, a likely prominent effect being the inhibition of mitochondrial oxidation (Ozawa *et al.* 1983). The hypermetabolic response to sepsis is described on page 11.

The outlook for patients with septic complications of gastrointestinal surgery has probably been transformed by the availability of parenteral and enteral nutrition, but verification of this opinion by clinical trials is neither practical nor ethical. In this chapter pragmatic guidelines are given towards maintaining nutritional requirements in the septic state.

Glucose

Studies of the oxidation of glucose in patients with sepsis have been contradictory and it has been suggested that wide variations in the clinical condition may explain the discrepancies observed. More recent data indicate a remarkable similarity of glucose utilization in septic patients with increase in the rate of gluconeogenesis (see p. 165), which is not completely suppressed by glucose infusion,

160

and in the absence of evidence of failure of glucose oxidation (Shaw *et al.* 1985). As in burns patients, high rates of glucose infusion for a prolonged period gives increased risk of fatty liver, hence a maximum glucose infusion rate of 5 mg/kg/minute is recommended.

The use of insulin (see p. 104) may enhance the protein sparing effect of glucose and improve the haemodynamic status of patients with septic shock (Bronsveld *et al.* 1985); its use is recommended to maintain blood glucose concentrations within the range 5–10 mmol/1.

Lipid

Patients with sepsis use lipid as a fuel. Using lipid to provide 50% or more of the energy supply achieves a similar degree of protein sparing in sepsis as a regime providing all non-protein energy as glucose (Baker *et al.* 1984). A regimen with lipid providing a maximum of 50% of non-protein calories is a practical recommendation.

Some patients may have a delayed lipid clearance and this should be checked for. The possibility that a lipid emulsion can give microemboli formation in acutely ill patients has been reported although the pathological significance of this observation is unclear; a test of this may be useful whereby small aliquots of patients serum and lipid emulsion are mixed and microscopically examined for evidence of clumping (Hulman *et al.* 1982).

Amino-acids

A major feature of sepsis is muscle protein breakdown and severe nitrogen loss. A characteristic plasma amino-acid pattern occurs early in the development of sepsis with, in particular, decreased levels of gluconeogenic and branched chain amino-acids (Roth *et al.* 1985).

For patients with sepsis, nutritional regimes enriched with branched chain amino-acids have been recommended but the evidence of improved protein sparing is so far suggestive rather than confirmatory (Sax *et al.* 1986). Biopsy measurements in sepsis have shown low hepatic and high muscle intracellular levels of branched chain amino-acids thus it may be that enhanced administration of these amino-acids in sepsis may benefit the metabolic requirements of liver rather than muscle.

Nitrogen administration of 0.25 g/kg/day is a practical recommendation.

Vitamins, Minerals

The requirements of these nutrients are comparable to those of other hypermetabolic conditions.

REFERENCES

Baker JP, Detsky AS, Stewarts S *et al.* (1984) TPN in the critically ill. *Gastroenterology*, **87**, 53–59.

Bronsveld W, Vanden Bos GC, Thijs L (1985) Use of glucose-insulin-potassium in human septic shock. *Critical Care Medicine*, **13**, 566–570.

Elubatc EA, Stoner HB (1983) The grading of sepsis. *B. J. Surg*, **70**, 29–31.

Hulman G, Fraser I, Pearson HJ *et al.* (1982) Agglutination of Intralipid by sera of acutely ill patients. *Lancet*, **ii**, 1426–1427.

Ozawa K, Aoyama H, Yasuda K *et al.* (1983) Metabolic abnormalities associated with postoperative organ failure. *Arch Surg*, **118**, 1245–1251.

Roth E, Mühlbacker F, Karner J *et al.* (1985) Liver amino-acids in sepsis. *Surgery*, **97**, 436–442.

Sax HP, Talamini M, Fischer J (1986) Clinical use of branched chain amino-acids in liver disease, sepsis, trauma and burns. *Arch Surg*, **121**, 358–366.

Shaw JH, Klein S, Wolfe RR (1985) Assessment of alanine, urea, and glucose interrelationships in normal subjects and in patients with sepsis. *Surgery*, **97**, 557–567.

Stevens LE (1985) Guaging the severity of surgical sepsis. *Arch Surg*, **118**, 1190–92.

Chapter 16 · Substrate Requirements in Burn Patients

A severe thermal burn initially causes loss of plasma and red blood cells. Following restoration of circulating blood volume, an increase in metabolic rate, hyperglycaemia and increased urinary nitrogen excretion occur. The hypermetabolic response in the burned patient is similar to other forms of injury but in the case of an extensive (> 30% body surface area) burn is often of greater magnitude and duration. Increased metabolic demands are made by tissue necrosis, loss of red blood cells, hyperthermia, multiple skin graft procedures and the development of infection. Following initial resuscitation nutritional support is started, usually by both enteral and parenteral routes when large amounts of fluid and calories are required.

Calorie requirements

The metabolic rate in the patient with a > 30% body surface area burn is on average 50–60% above the basal metabolic rate for the patient's particular age, sex and surface area (Fig. 16.1). The use of a high environmental temperature (Barr *et al.* 1968) and the early excision and closure of major burns (Burke *et al.* 1978) has probably helped to reduce very high metabolic rates.

A nutritional regimen which provides twice the basal metabolic requirements, together with adequate protein intake will result in positive nitrogen balance and prevent weight loss in most patients with extensive burns.

Glucose requirements

High (> 10 mg/kg/min) rates of glucose infusion are not energy efficient and do not result in further increases in glucose oxidation (Fig. 16.2). Excess glucose intake may be detrimental causing

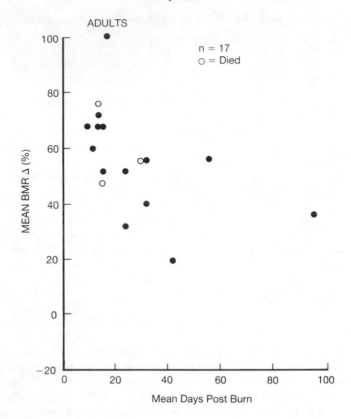

Fig. 16.1. Percentage increase in metabolic rate of adult burn patients admitted to the Massachusetts General Hospital.

carbon dioxide retention and hepatic lipid deposition (Burke *et al.* 1979). A glucose infusion of 4 mg/kg/min will suppress 70% of endogenous glucose production in the severely burned patient (Wolfe *et al.* 1979) and thus a glucose infusion rate of 5–7 mg/kg/min is probably ideal for both calorie requirements and avoiding glucose-induced morbidity. Insulin may be required to prevent hyperglycaemia and glycosuria when glucose in infused at high rates.

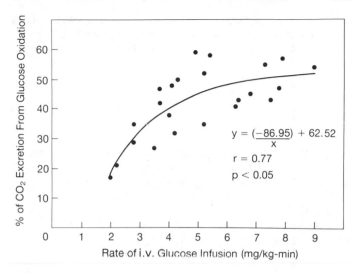

Fig. 16.2. Rate of glucose infusion and rate of glucose oxidation (kindly reproduced from the *Annals of Surgery*).

Protein requirements

Severe thermal injury causes large (10–25 g/24h) losses of urinary nitrogen and also losses of nitrogen through the wound (up to 0.1 g nitrogen/kg/day). Increased urinary nitrogen losses are the result of the difference between protein synthesis and catabolism, both of whose rates may be increased in severe burns (Kien *et al.* 1978). The optimum daily protein and amino acid requirements in burn patients are unknown but 300–500 mg nitrogen/kg Ideal Body Weight/day will usually result in a positive nitrogen balance.

Fat requirements

It has been shown that insulin and glucose can reduce nitrogen excretion in burned patients. A mixed regimen of glucose, fat and protein has however advantages and will result in a positive nitrogen balance. Lipid infusions provide essential fatty acids, can act as a medium for parenteral administration of fat-soluble vitamins and lessen both volume of water and the amount of glucose required. The latter is particularly of value in the treatment of young children with major burns. The optimum amount of fat required for burn patients is unknown but is unlikely to be greater than 50% of the non-protein calories supplied.

The formula currently used for calculating glucose, lipid and protein requirements in burns patients at the Massachusetts General Hospital is as follows:

Nitrogen requirements = 320 mgN/kg Ideal Body Weight/day
Total calories required = (Basal Metabolic Rate)* × 2
Calories from glucose = 5 mg/kg/min
Calories from lipid = Total calories − (glucose calories + protein calories†)

This results in a positive nitrogen balance in the great majority of children and adults with severe burns.

Delivery of parenteral feeding in burn patients

This is similar to other patients except that subcutaneously tunnelled central venous catheters can rarely be used in patients with major burns as the overlying skin may be required as a donor site. Catheters should be inserted through unbroken skin if possible and scrupulous care of the catheter is required to reduce the incidence of infection. Infection remains the commonest cause of death in burn patients (Sevitt 1979).

Monitoring nutritional support

In general this is similar to other patients. Hyperglycaemia is however common (Wolfe *et al.* 1979) and blood glucose concentration should be frequently measured. Anthropometric measurements are often impossible in the severely burned patient and falls in plasma albumin concentration may reflect the loss of albumin

*Obtained from appendix, p. 224.
†protein calories = gN × 25.

through open wounds or infection rather than malnutrition (Royle & Kettlewell 1980). Measurement of nitrogen balance still remains the best method of monitoring nutritional support in the severely burned patient; and prevention of weight loss and rate of recovery a guide to the effectiveness of treatment.

REFERENCES

Barr PO, Birke G, Liljedahl SO & Plantin L.O (1968) Oxygen consumption and water loss during treatment of burns with warm dry air. *Lancet*, i, 164–8.

Burke JF, Quinby WC & Bondoc CC (1978) Early excision and prompt wound closure supplemented with immunosuppression. In Symposium on Burns, *Surg Clin North Am*, **58**, 1141–50.

Burke JF, Wolfe RR, Mullany CJ, Mathews DE & Bier DM (1979) Glucose requirements following burn injury: Parameters of optimal glucose infusion and possible hepatic and respiratory abnormalities following excessive glucose intake. *Ann Surg*, **190**, 274–285.

Hinton P, Allison SP, Littlejohn S & Lloyd J (1971) Insulin and glucose to reduce the catabolic response to injury in burned patients. *Lancet*, i, 767–768.

Kien CL, Young VR, Rohrbaugh DK & Burke JF (1978) Increased rates of whole body protein synthesis and breakdown in children recovering from burns. *Ann Surg*, **187**, 383–391.

Royle GT & Kettlewell MGW (1980) Liver function tests in surgical infection and malnutrition. *Ann Surg*, **192**, 192–4.

Sevitt S (1979) A review of the complications of burns, their origin and importance for illness and death. *J Trauma*, **19**, 358–69.

Wolfe RR, Durkot MJ, Allsop JR, Burke JF (1979) Glucose metabolism in severely burned patients. *Metabolism*, **28**, 1031–39.

Chapter 17 · Parenteral Nutrition for Infants and Children

NUTRITIONAL REQUIREMENTS

Paediatric and adult parenteral feeding differ in two fundamental respects; firstly, the daily requirements of energy and nutrients change rapidly with age particularly in early infancy, and secondly, the daily allowance of energy and nutrients must cover not only basal requirements but also allow for growth. Parenteral feeds should therefore be complete and individual. Quantities should not only be adjusted to cover normal requirements but also to compensate for previous deficiencies and estimated further losses.

Energy: Adequate energy intake should cover basal metabolic requirements, physical activity and growth (see Table 17.1). Energy requirements may increase with illness, (see Table 17.2) and fall with reduced physical activity. In infancy and childhood the daily weight increase is a reasonable measure of energy sufficiency.

Energy sources: Many non-protein energy sources have been tried but only glucose and fat are now widely used (see Chapters 2 and

Table 17.1.

| | Energy expenditure/kg body weight/day | | | |
Age	Maintenance kcal (MJ) %	Growth kcal (MJ) %	Activity kcal (MJ) %	Total kcal (MJ)
birth—2 weeks	69(0.29) 66	26(0.1) 25	10(0.04) 9	105(0.43)
2 weeks—3/12	79(0.33) 66	28(0.12) 24	12(0.04) 10	119(0.49)
9/12—12/12	83(0.35) 79	6(0.03) 6	16(0.06) 15	105(0.44)
2 yrs—3 yrs	75(0.31) 75	2(0.01) 2	23(0.10) 23	100(0.42)
4 yrs—5 yrs	69(0.29) 70	2(0.01) 2	28(0.11) 28	99(0.41)
9 yrs—10 yrs	56(0.23) 73	1(0.004) 1.3	20(0.09) 26	77(0.32)
16 yrs—17 yrs	41(0.17) 80	1(0.004) 2	9(0.04) 18	51(0.21)

(World Health Organization, 1973 Energy and protein requirements, *WHO Technical report series*, **522**).

Table 17.2. Effect of illness on energy requirements

	(% increase over basal requirements)
Fever	12% for each degree above 37°C
Cardiac failure	15–25%
Major surgery	20–30%
Burns	up to 100%
Severe sepsis	40–50%
Long term growth failure	50–100%
Protein calorie malnutrition	36% + depending on age

(Kerner JA Jr. (ed) *Manual of pediatric parenteral nutrition* John Wiley & Sons, New York, 1976)

9). The equivalent osmolality and calorific values of varying glucose concentrations and fat emulsions are shown in Table 17.3). Although complications associated with the infusion of fat emulsion have been described, of which fat embolism in the pulmonary and cerebral circulation and cholestatic jaundice are the most relevant, to achieve a volume for volume energy equivalent with glucose alone entails the use of 25–50% solutions. The increase in osmolality of solutions as the concentration of glucose increases, however, rapidly becomes unacceptable in infants and young children. In addition, the infusion of excess quantities of glucose above that required to meet the basal metabolic rate and for synthesis of lean body tissue have been shown to produce fatty liver and increase carbon dioxide production (Askanazi *et al.* 1980; Burke *et al.* 1979). Burke *et al.* (1979) have also suggested that glucose utilization plateaus at 5 mg/kg/min, but children and neonates in particular may utilize higher infusion rates. It therefore seems reasonable to use a combination of fat and glucose to supply energy requirements.

Table 17.3. Energy sources: Osmolality and Calorific values (approximate)

Fat emulsion	10%	250 mOsm/kg	1 kcal/ml	
Fat emulsion	20%	300 mOsm/kg	2 kcal/ml	
Glucose	5%	277 mOsm/kg	0.2 kcals/ml	200 kcals/l
Glucose	10%	555 mOsm/kg	0.4 kcals/ml	400 kcals/l
Glucose	20%	1110 mOsm/kg	0.8 kcals/ml	
Glucose	50%	2775 mOsm/kg	2 kcals/ml	

Glucose tolerance in sick children and premature infants in particular is poor. Insulin infusions may therefore be needed to improve carbohydrate tolerance and facilitate weight gain. Infusions of 0.01 to 0.02 u/kg/hour appear satisfactory but require individual monitoring. Insulin should be mixed in the glucose infusion to avoid hypoglycaemia if the infusion is inadvertently discontinued.

Fluid requirements

The fluid volume available will to some extent influence the choice of intravenous solutions and should be calculated first. Maintenance fluid requirements change with age (see below) and additional fluid may be needed to replace excess losses from diarrhoea, high output ostomies or with fever. Since parenteral feeding is not an emergency procedure, dehydration and gross electrolyte disturbances should be corrected before feeding is started.

Maintenance fluid requirements:

1 infants up to 10 kg — 0–6 months 150 ml/kg/day
                          6–12 months 110 ml/kg/day
2 child of wt > 10 kg — 1000 ml for first 10 kg
                          500 ml for next 10 kg
                          20 ml for each additional kg

Fluid requirement can also be estimated in relation to energy intake:

1.5 ml/kcal (360 ml/MJ) for infants < 10 kg
1.0–1.25 ml/kcal (240–300 ml/MJ) for older children.

Amino acid requirements

The ideal amino acid profile for parenteral feeding in infants and children is yet to be derived. Not only are the overall protein requirements higher in children, (see Table 17.4) but individual amino acid requirements vary with age. In addition to the eight amino acids described as essential in adults (p. 21), histidine appears essential in infants (Snyderman *et al*. 1963). Cystine and tyrosine (Gaull *et al*. 1972) may also be required in the premature

Table 17.4. Protein requirements

	Age	Median weight (kg)	Protein intake (g/kg)	(g/day) *
Months	3–6	7	1.85	13
	6–9	8.5	1.65	14
	9–12	9.5	1.50	14
Years	1–2	11	1.20	13.5
	2–3	13.5	1.15	15.5
	3–5	16.5	1.10	17.5
	5–7	20.5	1.0	21
	7–10	27	1.0	27

* (rounded to nearest 0.5 g) requirement may be higher in illness.

Calorie/nitrogen ratio for nitrogen accumulation: 150–250 non protein kcal/g nitrogen.

(WHO 1985 Energy and Protein Requirements. Report of a Joint FAO/WHO/UNU Expert Consultation World Health Organization Technical Report Series No. 724).

infant. Taurine may also be necessary for optimal hepatic function and development of the retina, CNS and cardiac muscle in premature infants (Gaull *et al.* 1977) although studies using taurine supplemented feeds have given equivocal results.

In the absence of an ideal formulation, amino acid solutions with a profile based on a first class protein model such as egg or more recently breast milk have been used. Overall these appear to give satisfactory results, however intravenous solutions based on the amino acid profiles of oral feeds fail to take into account the effect of gut mucosal transaminases and may lead to imbalances with glutamic and aspartic acid. The use of amino acid solutions primarily developed for adults have also resulted in imbalances in blood amino acid levels which may produce growth retardation (Harper 1959) and hepatic dysfunction (Seashore 1980). Elevated phenylaline levels may be a particular problem in preterm infants. The use of transfer adapted solutions may overcome this problem, but, as yet, experience with these solutions in children is limited. Solutions containing high concentrations of glycine are best avoided in view of the effect on the renal tubular resorption of proline and serine (Kellerman *et al.* 1976). The amino acid contents of commonly available solutions are shown on page 227, of these only Vamin 9 contains cystine and appears suitable for use in infants and young children. Other solutions may be satisfactory in older children.

Indications for intravenous fat

Certain polyunsaturated fatty acids (linoleic acid) are essential components of cell membranes and deficiency leads to clinical problems (Table 17.5). Fatty acid deficiency can be prevented in adults by lipolysis of endogenous adipose tissue, however fat reserves in the small infant are meagre, and biochemical evidence of fatty acid deficiency has been noted in the serum of neonates as early as two days after starting TPN, (Friedman *et al.* 1976) and clinical signs and symptoms within 28 days. Biochemical evidence of fatty acid deficiency is a triene/tetraene ratio >0.4 (ratio of eicosatrienoic to arachidonic acid). The amount of dietary linoleic acid found to prevent both clinical and biochemical deficiency is 1–2% of dietary calories. Essential fatty acid deficiency may also be prevented in patients not on complete bowel rest with oral fat solutions (corn or sunflower seed oil, 30 ml in divided doses). The benefits of cutaneous applications of essential fatty acid rich oils have not been conclusively proven (Hunt *et al.* 1978).

Fat metabolism

Intravenously administered fat has a similar metabolic pathway to that of naturally occurring chylomicrons. Clearance from the bloodstream is dependant on lipoprotein-lipase activity. This enzymatic hydrolysis of circulating bound triglyceride occurs at

Table 17.5. Signs and symptoms of fatty acid deficiency.

Growth retardation
Dermatitis
Hair loss
Poor wound healing
Thrombocytopoenia
Increased erythrocyte fragility
Decreased immuno competence

capillary endothelium in muscle and adipose tissue. Lipid clearance from plasma is accelerated in catabolic states, and with the concurrent use of heparin, glucose or insulin.

Complications associated with fat infusions (see p. 116)

If the rate of fat infusion exceeds the clearance rate, hyperlipidaemia occurs and the plasma becomes turbid. Advisable infusion rates are given in Tables 17.10 and 17.11, however considerable variation in tolerance is seen and levels must be monitored in the individual patient. Visual inspection of plasma for turbidity is unreliable for monitoring intravenous fat accumulation and preferred methods are nephelometry:- levels < 100–150 mg/dl (Forget *et al.* 1975), or biochemical determination of plasma triglycerides, cholesterol and fatty acids.

Altered pulmonary function

Conflicting data exist on the effect of fat infusions on pulmonary diffusing capacity and arterial oxygen tension and saturation. Pulmonary fat accumulation has also been described after infusions of 20% fat emulsion in very low birth weight infants (Levene *et al.* 1980). These effects appear related to excessive infusion rates (>0.15 g/kg/hour) which are particularly likely if attempting to 'catch up' lost fluid volumes after drip resiting and should be avoided.

Impaired immunity

Fischer *et al.* (1980) have shown impaired bacterial clearance following intraperitoneal injections of fat emulsion in mice and inhibition of chemotaxis in human neutrophils *in vitro* following preincubation in emulsion. More recent studies have failed to confirm these observations (English *et al.* 1981).

Jaundice

Of particular importance in paediatric practice is the displacement of bilirubin from albumin by free fatty acids released from the hydrolysis of infused fat emulsions. This may increase the risk of kernicterus (Thiessein *et al.* 1972). Kerner (1983) has shown that a continuous fat infusion over 20 hours, started during the second week of life when the bilirubin level was less than half the potential exchange level for the individual patient did not increase the risk of kernicterus.

Vitamins

Multivitamin solutions suitable for paediatric use are shown in the appendix (p. 233). Although oral recommended daily vitamin intakes (pp. 198–9) can serve as a general guide, these recommendations have to be modified for TPN use and requirements are generally higher. Water-soluble vitamins delivered systemically have a higher renal clearance than oral vitamins, and photodegradation and binding to infusion apparatus is likely to occur (Allwood 1984).

Specific requirements

Vitamin C is a necessary cofactor in premature infants because of diminished hepatic tyrosine transaminase activity (Gordon *et al.* 1944). Deficiency of biotin and fat-soluble vitamins are particularly likely in children with short gut syndromes or those receiving continuous antibiotics which suppress intestinal flora. The Vitamin D content of the multivitamin solutions is inadequate for premature infants where an intake in excess of 10 μg/day is needed. Simply increasing the amount of multivitamin solution may risk hypervitaminosis A, extra Vitamin D should therefore be added separately, as alfacalcidol injection (Leo Laboratories).

Trace elements

Trace elements play a major part in the synthesis and structural stabilization of proteins and nucleic acids. They are also constituents of hormones. Although there are few data on amounts

Table 17.6. Daily trace element requirements

Element	Infants + Children < 20 kg* dosage/kg/day	> 20 kg total dosage	Premature infants† dose/kg/day
Iron	approx 1–1.5 mg/kg/day		12.6 μmol
Zinc	1.5 μmol	60 μmol	7.5 μmol
Copper	0.3 μmol	16 μmol	1.5 μmol
Manganese	0.12 μmol	15 μmol	140 nmol
Chromium	3 nmol	0.2 μmol	105 nmol

* to max dosage of 20 kg.
† James *et al.* 1979.

required, trace element deficiency states have been noted in infants receiving parenteral nutrition (Latimer *et al.* 1980), and supplements must therefore be regarded as essential. The daily requirements for infants and older children are shown in Table 17.6 together with calculated requirements for premature infants (James *et al.* 1979). Commercially available trace element solutions are shown in the appendix page 235. To avoid toxic accumulation trace element dosage should be reduced or omitted during the first week of life particularly in premature infants when renal function is poorly developed. The copper and manganese intakes must also be reduced in patients with obstructive jaundice since these metals are excreted in the bile.

The iron requirements of growing infants and children are not met by trace element solutions alone and incompatibilities and the risk of anaphylaxis limits the use of iron-dextran preparations, however additional iron may be supplied by 'top-up' transfusions.

The zinc intakes suggested in Table 17.6 may be inadequate, particularly in premature infants (Lockitch *et al.* 1983). Also amino acid solutions tend to form complexes with minerals, particularly zinc, and thereby induce often substantial urinary losses (Freeman *et al.* 1975). Both zinc and magnesium losses are also likely to increase with large volume losses of intestinal fluid.

Biochemical selenium deficiency is common with long-term feeding because of the low-selenium content of many commercial solutions. Symptomatic deficiency appears rare but individual monitoring and supplementation with doses 0.2 μmol/day (16 μg) (i.v.) appears safe and advisable.

INFUSION TECHNIQUES

Several important advances have occurred in delivery systems in recent years which have been of particular use in paediatric practice. The first has been the increasing availability of fine bore cannulae, and the second the development of volumetric infusion pumps.

Peripheral infusions

The use of peripheral veins is to be preferred in all ages to reduce infective complications. Even newborns can be managed for considerable periods in this way. Numerous fine cannulae (e.g. Jelco 22 Gauge) are available and are preferable to Butterfly needles. Methods of fixation are very much of personal preference but which ever method is used the region of the cannula or needle tip should be kept visible so that extravasation can be detected early. In this respect transparent adhesive dressings are particularly useful.

Many centres advocate changing peripheral drip-sites daily on the grounds that these veins may be re-useable at a later date.

Central venous catheters

These become necessary when all peripheral sites have been exhausted, however an elective change to a central line may help with mobilization since patients can be disconnected for variable periods by using a heparin lock. The use of central lines may also be preferable to long periods between drip resiting and consequent risk of hypoglycaemia. Whichever method of insertion is used strict aseptic technique is mandatory.

Percutaneous techniques

In newborns and infants fine silastic catheters can be introduced via scalp or arm veins but the technique is difficult as is fixation. At present we are generally using the subclavian or internal jugular routes with the patient anaesthetized. The Vygon Leader-Cath (code 115.09) utilizes a 20 G. needle and a Seldinger wire for insertion. However, the manufacturers advise removal after seven days because of 'leaching' of plasticisers and hardening of the cannula. The same company's 'Desilet' system (1129.04) enables a silicone catheter (Nutricath S—code 2180.20) to be introduced, again using only a 20 G. needle. The Nutricath has the advantage of an excellent adapter for connecting the silicone catheter to a Luer fitting.

In older children many systems are available for introducing long-line catheters via peripheral veins. The Desilet system mentioned above is available in a number of sizes and is as good as any. The cephalic vein in the antecubital fossa is commonly used but has the disadvantage of immobilizing the arm.

Operative techniques

Where feeding may be anticipated to last for many weeks or months we are currently using the Broviac or Hickman silastic catheters (Schuco International Ltd, Cat. Nos. EV 201, 204, 206, outside diameters 1.4–3.2 mm). This catheter has a dacron cuff attached which lies just inside the skin entry site and ensures firm fixation by fibrous tissue. In newborns the size of the catheter means using large veins such as the internal jugular for access but in older children the cephalic vein in the delto-pectoral groove is usually of sufficient size. This type of catheter is in use for patients on home i.v. feeding. Similar catheters are available from other manufacturers (e.g. Vygon Life-Vac & Life-Cath range). Multiple lumen catheters may be useful where multiple infusions are required via the same access site (e.g. concurrent parenteral nutrition plus cytotoxic therapy).

Delivery systems

Volumetric infusion pumps are now available which will deliver

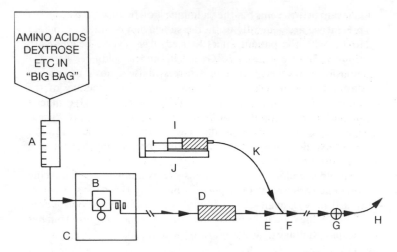

Fig. 17.1. Intravenous feeding mixtures are provided pre-mixed in a collapsible bag, and fat emulsions are supplied in pre-filled syringes. The burette is used as a check on the volumetric accuracy of the pump. For intravenous additives (e.g. antibiotics): a, infusions are given proximal to the filter D by including a connector (as E) and suitable administration apparatus; b, small volume injections are given distal to the filter using the integral injection port. Such injections are drawn into the syringe through a 5 μm filter needle (Argyle 8881305018) to remove particles. The volume of tubing between this injection port and the catheter is approximately 2 ml. This must be flushed or allowed for when timing administration and blood sampling for monitoring drugs such as gentamicin.

Key: A, Burette administration set (non-vented). [Soluset 1876 (Abbott) or A200/A2000 (Avon)]; B, IMED cassette (C924); C, IMED volumetric pump, Model 922 or 960 with air-in-line detector; D, Filter, air eliminating, 0.2 μm; [Ultipor FAE-020-LYL (Pall) or Cathivex SVGS 025 YS (Millipore)] with injection port below filter; E, Connector or one-way valve with connector; [889.00 or 284.00 (Vygon)]. (Valve in line with filter); F, Tubing with small internal diameter, long; [Lectrocath (Vygon) 1155.20]; G, One-way tap, permanently attached to catheter; [872.10 (Vygon)]; H, Catheter (short piece of tubing attached to bring tap outside clothing if necessary); I, Syringe, 60 ml with fat emulsion; [BD Plastipak]; J, Syringe pump, Vickers Treonic IP3 or IP4; K, Tubing with small internal diameter, short; [Lectroflex (Vygon) 222.02].

Note
1 All connections should be 'Luer Lock'
2 G & H are assembled in theatre when catheter placed. All apparatus down to, but not including, the tap (G) is replaced daily
3 If larger amounts of fat are administered from a bottle the syringe pump is replaced with a volumetric pump and suitable apparatus
4 If an all-in-one mixture including fat is used the filter is omitted.

fluids accurately to within 0.1 ml. There are also available a number of 0.2 micron air-venting filters which remove particulate matter from the i.v. solutions, prevent air-embolism and possibly inhibit bacterial contamination. Figures 17.1–17.4 show the complete infusion assembly; microbore tubing is used wherever possible with luer locks for all connections. An opaque plastic cover is used to cover the feed bag to prevent photo degradation of the multivitamin solution used in the intravenous feed. For neonates, where the solution may remain in a burette for long periods, it may be desirable to use apparatus which reduces photodegradation (e.g. Avon A2000 Ultra-Violet Filter Solution Burette set and tubing).

Preparation of solutions

These should be prepared in the pharmacy using conditions discussed in Chapter 3.

To simplify administration the components of the regimen should be packed in a single, sterile, collapsible bag container. The amount of calcium infused in young children may produce com-

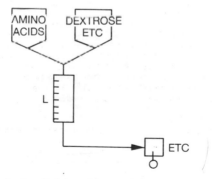

Fig. 17.2. Alternative if amino acid solutions and dextrose solutions are not supplied pre-mixed.
Key: L, Twin lead burette [A202 (Avon)] or triple lead burette [(C)788 (Travenol)]
Note
1 These burettes do not have shut-off valves
2 Air inlet sets required with bottles

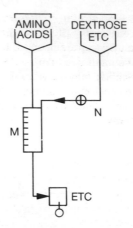

Fig. 17.3. Alternative to Fig. 17.2 if special burettes not available or if shut-off valve considered essential. Key: M, Burette administration set (vented). [Soluset 1882 (Abbott)] N, Plasma transfer set. [C2240 (Travenol)]
Note:
1 Latex plug of burette is removed aseptically and N plugged in

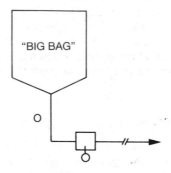

Fig. 17.4. Alternative if frequent re-filling of burette is to be avoided e.g. home i.v. feeding. Key: O, IMED cassette (C924-QNV). (Has integral administration set) OR Solution administration set (Luer-Lock). [CO334 (Travenol)] attached to IMED cassette (C924).

patibility problems with added phosphate and fat emulsion. Most standard requirements of calcium, phosphate and amino acids can be included in the same mixture if the child is not fluid restricted. However, formulations should be carefully checked and if necessary calcium and phosphate may be administered on alternate days. It may be possible to add fat emulsion to the mixtures. Compatibility and stability of solutions in 3 litre bags have been reviewed by Allwood (1984).

Compounding

Bags of varying sizes (250, 500 ml, 1 l, 2 l, 3 l) are available in PVC and EVA. Larger bags will have transfer sets attached allowing traditional gravity or vacuum transfer of solutions. However, this is only suitable for whole-bottle quantities and therefore applicable to older children and adolescents. Neonates and infants require more accurate transfer of volumes than these techniques allow.

Burette and syringe transfer techniques are available using commercial or home produced equipment. If large numbers of patients are dealt with an automated transfer device such as the Automix (Travenol) is required. This allows up to three solutions to be rapidly pumped into a sterile container. Volume is calculated from specific gravity of the solutions keyed into a microprocessor and the weight transferred which is detected by a load cell. Accuracy of fluid transfer is claimed to be $\pm 5\%$ for volumes > 250 ml and ± 15 ml for volumes < 250 ml.

The chief disadvantage of this equipment is its cost of about £8000.

Administration of solutions

Full aseptic technique must be used when assembling administration equipment and attaching feeding solutions (see Chapter 4). It may be possible to attach equipment to the feeding container when it is prepared in the pharmacy.

If possible the equipment used for administering feeding

solutions should not be used for the injection or infusion of other drugs. However, in infants and children it may only be possible to get venous access at one site. In this case the compatibility of drugs with feeding solutions must be checked or the line flushed with saline prior to administration. In neonates this may lead to administration of excessive quantities of fluid and requires careful control.

In general drugs should be injected proximal to the 0.2 μm filter. With small doses of some drugs, however, loss to the filter may be considerable. These should be injected distal to the filter with the tubing between injection site and filter clamped shut. Drugs should be drawn into the syringe through a filter needle (Argyle 8881305018) to remove particles. When monitoring blood levels of injected drugs it is important to take into account the volume of tubing (between injection site and vein) in relation to solution flow rate. Small bore tubing and a filter with low dead space must be used. Human albumin solutions may be infused through the 0.2 μm filter but fresh plasma and similar blood products must not. The calcium content of feeding solutions may produce coagulation of fresh plasma if co-administered.

THE PRETERM INFANT

In the UK approximately 7% of all newborns weigh < 2.5 kg, of these one third are dysmature (i.e. weight < 10% for their gestational age) and two-thirds are premature (born before 37 weeks of gestation). Improved methods of intensive care can now offer even the most premature a better than 50% chance of survival. This and the increasing use of surgery in the newborn has created a need for safe and efficient parenteral nutrition in infants weighing only a few hundred grams.

The fluid, energy and nitrogen requirements in the premature infant are uncertain and likely to be modified by stress, sepsis and environmental factors. Complex changes also occur in cardio-respiratory, hepatic and renal function and skin permeability after birth that may influence these requirements.

Table 17.7. Period of survival during starvation

	Starvation/days	Semi-starvation/days
Adult	100	365
Term infant	32	80
Premature infant (2.0 kg)	12	30
Premature infant (1.0 kg)	4	10

(Heird *et al. J Pediatr* 1972, **80**, 351–372).

Indications for i.v. feeding

The nutritional reserves of a neonate at term are poor compared with the adult (Table 17.7) and are even more limited in the premature infant. The neonatal period is also a time of rapid growth and development. Experimental evidence suggests that inadequate nutrition when tissues are undergoing rapid cell division results in a reduction in body DNA and also in brain DNA content (Davidson & Dobbin 1968; Winick & Rosso 1969). Since glial proliferation in the human brain is accelerating during the last trimester of pregnancy, preterm infants are likely to be particularly vulnerable to the effects of malnutrition. This resulting cell loss cannot be made up by 'catch up' growth as is seen in later childhood. Failure, therefore to establish oral feeds by day 4 is an indication for parenteral feeding.

Fluid balance

More than 90% of a 26 week foetus is water, of which 50% is represented by the extracellular fluid, these proportions fall progressively with age. The exact fluid requirements are often difficult to assess and likely to be modified by variations in transepidermal loss and renal function. The premature kidney has only a limited ability to excrete a water load and with glomerular development preceding tubular function, high urinary sodium losses occur (Siegel & Oh 1976). Precise fluid management is therefore important. Too rapid infusions (> 150 ml/kg) are associated with symptomatic patent ductus arteriosis (Bell *et al.* 1980) and necrotizing enterocolitis (Bell *et al.* 1979), too slow an infusion (< 120 ml/kg) can rapidly lead to dehydration because of high insensible fluid losses (Oh 1982). Additional fluid losses can result from hyperglycaemia, with each mmol increase in blood glucose concentration producing an increase in serum osmolality of 1 mOsm/1 and an osmotic diuresis (Brans 1977).

In view of the small fluid volumes used in this group of patients all fluids given or lost should be considered in the daily balance. Slow infusions to maintain venous or arterial access for drugs or gas sampling represent wasted fluid volume. Drugs should be given in minimal fluid volumes and repeated flushing of intravenous lines after injections or infusion can contribute a significant fluid load. Similarly repeated blood sampling represents a sizeable loss and can rapidly lead to anaemia. Haemoglobins in these infants should be maintained above 13.5 g/dl by transfusions of packed cells.

Daily fluid requirements can be estimated from the table of insensible fluid losses given below (Table 17.8), together with measured fluid losses in urine and stools and or daily weight change in conjunction with the clinical condition.

Radiant heat warmers increase the insensible water loss (IWL) by 50–100% in infants < 1500 g compared with incubators and by 82–190% in infants > 1500 g. Phototherapy increases IWL in infants < 1500 g by 81% and in infants > 1500 g by 192%. This can be reduced to 42% in < 1500 g infants and to 113% in infants > 1500 g by maintaining the skin temperature at 36.5°C by servo control.

Table 17.8. Changes in insensible water loss (IWL) with weight and post gestational age

Weight in g	IWL ml/kg/24 hr	Week 1	Week 2	Week 3	Week 4
< 1000	64				
1001–1250	56	57	50	41	38
1251–1500	38				
1501–1750	22	20	32	30	30
1751–2000	17				

(figures for well infants in servo incubators at 35% relative humidity).

(Wu & Hodgman 1974 *Pediatr* **54**, 704–712).

Energy requirements: the cost of growth

The last trimester of pregnancy is a period of rapid growth and development, with the average fetus doubling in weight from 1000 to 2000 g between 27 and 32 weeks. During that time 120 g of protein, 120 g of fat and 10 g of minerals are deposited. To achieve this growth requires energy, both in terms of stored energy, i.e. deposited fat and protein and energy for tissue synthesis. The latter is approximately 7.5 kcal/g for protein and 11.6 kcal/g for fat. Energy is also required for resting body metabolism, thermo-regulation and activity (see Table 17.9). The energy input needed to achieve the rate of accretion seen in utero is rarely achievable using either parenteral or enteral feeding or any combination of the two because of the premature infant's poor glucose and fat tolerance and a limited ability to excrete a water load. In this situation of suboptimal energy intake, basal requirements will be met at the cost of growth.

Minimizing energy losses

Since energy intake is at a premium it is imperative to minimize all energy losses to allow the maximum use of calories for growth. The 'tiny' baby has a comparatively high surface area relative to its volume from which it can lose heat. The inability to reduce this exposed surface area by assuming a flexed posture and the lack of an insulative layer of subcutaneous fat leads to immense heat losses. Evaporation from the permeable skin also results in heat

Table 17.9. Energy requirements in preterm infants

		kcal/kg/day
Expenditure	resting metabolism	50
	activity	10
	thermo regulation	10
	tissue synthesis	25) energy cost
Storage		25) of growth
Total		120

Brooke OG (1982) *Br J Hosp Med*, **28**, 462–469.

loss. The increased metabolic rate that results in cold-stressed infants leads to rapid depletion of hepatic glycogen and possible hypoglycaemia. Heat losses can be minimized by nursing in a thermo-neutral environment. Reduction in air currents by the use of plastic films, minimal handling and limiting evaporation by coating the skin with paraffin are simple, cheap and effective means of reducing energy requirements.

Practical guidelines

1　Suitable feeding regimens for infants and children are given in Table 17.10 and for low birth weight infants in Table 17.11. Delivery systems are illustrated in Figs. 17.1–17.4.

2　Carbohydrates are introduced in a stepwise fashion to allow appropriate endogenous insulin response and thus prevent hyper-glycaemia and subsequent osmotic diuresis. Glucose tolerance is particularly poor in premature infants so the carbohydrate intake should be calculated in g/kg/day rather than 5% or 10% glucose solutions given at rates to meet fluid requirements.

3　Rebound hypoglycaemia is likely if infusions are abruptly ter-minated, drips should therefore be resited promptly. If venous access is difficult and resiting causes delay, a change to a central line should be considered. Discontinuation of infusions should be tapered over several days as oral feeds are established.

4　Intravenous fat tolerance varies and requires monitoring in the individual patient. Attempts to 'catch-up' lost infusion volumes should not be made with fat emulsions. All infused solutions run concurrently, however, fat emulsions are stopped for 4 hours prior to blood sampling, rates should therefore be calculated over 20 hours. Intravenous fat will not infuse through the filters suggested in Fig. 17.1. Fat emulsions should not be given in neonates if the serum bilirubin $> \frac{1}{2}$ the exchange level.

5　To achieve efficient protein utilization 150–250 non-protein calories are required per g of nitrogen infused. Acidosis may occur in neonates with excessive amino acid infusions.

6　The excessive administration of chloride should be avoided by using potassium phosphate, calcium gluconate or sodium acetate

Table 17.10. Average daily intravenous requirements

		1.5–2.5 kg	< 10 kg	10–30 kg	> 30 kg
Water	ml/kg	See fluid requirements page 170			
Calories	kcal/kg	110–115	120	75	50
Non protein kcal/gN		250	200–250	150–200	150
Protein	g/kg	2.5–3.1	2.5	2.0	1.5
Nitrogen	g/kg	0.4–0.5	0.4	0.3	0.2
Fat (< 4 g/kg/day)		< 40% of total calories		< 50% total calories	
Sodium	mmol/kg	3–5	2–5	2–3	2–3
Potassium	mmol/kg	2–3	2–3	2–3	2–3
Chloride	mmol/kg	2–4	2–5	2–4	2–4
Calcium	mmol/kg	0.5–1.0	0.5	0.5	0.25–0.5
Magnesium	mmol/kg	0.25	0.25	0.2	0.1
Phosphate	mmol/kg	0.25–0.5	0.25–0.5	0.1–0.4	0.1–0.2
Vitamins MVS		1 ml	2 ml	5 ml	5 ml
B12		50–100 µg monthly			
Folic acid		1 mg weekly		1 mg daily	1 mg daily
Vitamin K		0.5 mg twice weekly		1.0 mg twice weekly	5 mg twice weekly
Trace element solutions		Pedel 3 ml/kg per day to max of 30 ml		Addamel 0.25–0.5 ml/kg	

If Calcium and Magnesium cannot be mixed with Phosphate, double the daily dose requirements and alternate trace elements, Ca and Mg with Phosphate on successive days.

(Heparin 0.5–1.0 units/ml is added to minimise thrombosis and reduce catheter colonization. The effect on lipid clearance at this dosage is uncertain)

MVS – Multiple Vitamin Solution (IMS)

or bicarbonate. The concentration of divalant cations (calcium) needed in many paediatric feeding regimes precludes the mixing of fat with electrolyte solutions otherwise 'cracking' of the fat emulsion may occur. Precipitation may occur if large quantities of calcium and phosphate are mixed in small volumes in the same

Table 17.11. Parenteral feeding regime for very low birth weight neonates (<1.500 g) (Amount/kg/day).

Day of PN	Age (days)	Fluid vol	Glucose g	Nitrogen g	Nitrogen ml†	Fat 10% g	Fat 10% ml	Na	K	Ca	Mg	PO4
1	3	90	5	0.09	10	–	0	3–6	2–3	1	0.5	0.5
2		100	8	0.11	12	–	0	3–6	2–3	1	0.5	0.5
3		120	8	0.14	15	0.5	5	3–6	2–3	1	0.5	0.5
4		140	10	0.19	20	0.5	5	3–6	2–3	1	0.5	0.5
5		150	10	0.19	20	1.0	10	3–6	2–3	1	0.5	0.5
6		150	12	0.24	25	1.0	10	3–6	2–3	1	0.5	0.5
7 + over		150–200	15–24	0.28	30	2.0	20	3–6	2–3	1	0.5	0.5
Kcals			56–90	12 (non protein) 22								

Total kcals 90 cals/kg/day based on total feed of 150 ml/kg/day or 124 kcals/kg/day based on total feed of 200 ml/kg/day

†Vamin 9 Glucose; containing 9.4 g Nitrogen/litre in 10% dextrose (KabiVitrum Ltd.)

Vitamins

Folic acid	50 μg/day
B12	50 μg twice monthly
Vit K	0.25–0.5 mg twice weekly
MVS	1 ml/day

Trace elements

Pedel	4 ml/kg from 7th day

bag. Pedel provides 0.3 mmol phosphate/kg. The balance is added as sodium or potassium phosphates. Compatability should be checked. Alternate day infusion appears satisfactory but allowance must be made in interpretation of electrolyte results.

7   Trace element solutions should be avoided in premature infants for the first week of life, and infusions reduced in the presence of renal or hepatic failure.

8   Bacterial colonization of central lines appears more frequent in infants, with *staphylococcus albus* being the most frequent pathogen. A spiking temperature necessitates blood cultures and discontinuation of fat infusions. We have not found the clearing of lines by long-term antibiotic therapy alone successful, however

symptoms settle rapidly with catheter removal. Bacterial end\
carditis appears rare in the absence of cardiac anomolies.

9   Blocked catheters can be cleared using urokinase (Leo Laboratories) 5000 u in 2 ml of water. The solution is injected and gently agitated for 15 minutes before being withdrawn and the line heparinized for 45 minutes. This procedure can be repeated × 3 in a four hour period if the platelet count is > 20 000. This procedure is also used in combination with antibiotics to clear catheters colonized by *staphylococcus albus*.

10   Every attempt should be made to continue oral feeds, even in small volumes to improve endogenous insulin response and maintain the swallowing reflex.

REFERENCES

Allwood MC (1984) Compatibility and stability of TPN mixtures in big bags. *J Clin Hosp Pharm*, **9**, 181 198.

Askanazi J, Rosenbaum SH, Hyman AI, Silverberg PA, Milic-Emili J, & Kinney JM. (1980) Respiratory changes induced by the large glucose loads of total parenteral nutrition. *JAMA*, **243**, 1444 1447.

Bell EF, Warburton D, Stonestreet BS & Oh W (1980) Effect of fluid administration on the development of symptomatic patent ductus arteriosus and congestive heart failure in premature infants. *N Engl J Med*, **302**, 598-604.

Bell EF, Warburton D, Stonestreet BS *et al.* (1979) High volume fluid intake predisposes premature infants to necrotizing enterocolitis. *Lancet*, **ii**, 90.

Brans YW (1977) Parenteral nutrition of the very low birth weight neonate: a critical view. *Clin Perinatol*,**4**, 367.

Burke JF, Wolfe RR, Mullany CJ, Mathews DE & Bier DM (1979) Glucose requirements following burn injury. Parameters of optimal glucose infusion and possible hepatic and respiratory abnormalities following excessive glucose intake. *Ann Surg*, **190**, 274-285.

Davidson AN & Dobbin J (1968) The developing brain. Davidson AN and Dobbing J (eds) *Applied Neurochemistry*. Blackwell Scientific Publications, Oxford.

English D, Roloff JS, Lukens JN *et al.* (1981) Intravenous lipid emulsions and human neutrophil function. *J Pediat*, **99**,913-916.

Fischer GW, Hunter KW, Wilson SR & Mease AD (1980) Diminished bacterial defences with intralipid. *Lancet*, **ii**, 819-820.

Forget PP, Fernandes J & Begemann PH (1975) Utilization of fat emulsion during total parenteral nutrition in children. *Acta Paediat Scand*, **64**, 377-384.

Freeman JB, Stegink LD, Meyer PD, Fry LK & Denbesten L (1975) Excessive urinary zinc losses during parenteral alimentation. *J Surg Res*, **18**, 463-69.

Friedman Z, Danon A, Stahlman MT & Oates JA (1976) Rapid onset of essential fatty acid deficiency in the newborn. *Pediatr*, **58**, 640–649.

Gaull GE, Rassin DK, Raiha NCR & Heinonen K (1977) Milk protein quantity and quality in low birth weight infants III. Effects on sulfur amino acids in plasma and urine. *J Pediatr*, **90**, 348–355.

Gaull GE, Sturman JA & Raiha NCR (1972) Development of mammalian sulfur metabolism: absence of cystathionase in human fetal tissues. *Pediatr Res*, **6**, 538.

Gordon HH & Levine SZ (1944) The metabolic basis for the individualized feeding of infants, premature and full-term. *J Pediatr*, **25**, 464–475.

Harper AE (1959) Amino acid balance and imbalance. 1. Dietary level of protein and amino acid imbalance. *J Nutr*, **68**, 405–418.

Hunt CE, Engel RR, Modler S *et al.* (1978) Essential fatty acid deficiency in neonates: Inability to reverse deficiency by topical application of EFA-rich oil. *J Pediatrics*, **92**, 603–7.

James BE, Hendry PG & MacMahon RA (1979) Total parenteral nutrition of premature infants. 2. Requirement for micronutrient elements. *Aust Paediatr J*, **15**, 67–71.

Kellerman GM, MacMahon RA, Leber MH & James BE (1976) Amino acid studies during complete intravenous feeding of small premature infants. *Aust Paediat*, **12**, 255–260.

Kerner JA (Jr) ed. (1983) *Manual of pediatric parenteral nutrition.* John Wiley & Sons, New York.

Latimer JS, McClain CJ & Sharp HL (1980) Clinical zinc deficiency during zinc-supplemented parenteral nutrition. *J Pediatr*, **97**, 434–439.

Levene MI, Wigglesworth JS & Desai R (1980) Pulmonary fat accumulation after intralipid infusion in the preterm infant. *Lancet*, **ii**, 815–818.

Lockitch G, Godolphin W, Pendray MR *et al.* (1983) Serum zinc, copper, retinol-binding protein, prealbumin and ceruloplasmin concentrations in infants receiving intravenous zinc and copper supplementation. *J Pediatr*, **102**, 304–308.

Oh W. (1982) Fluid and electrolyte therapy and parenteral nutrition in low birth weight infants. *Clinics in Perinatology*, **9**, 637–643.

Seashore JH (1980) Metabolic complications of parenteral nutrition in infants and children. *Surgical Clinics of North America*. **60**, 1239–1252.

Siegel SR & Oh W (1976) Renal function as a marker of human fetal maturation. *Acta Paediat Scand*, **65**, 481–485.

Snyderman SE, Boyer A, Roitman E, Holt LE Jr & Prose PH (1963) The histidine requirement of the infant. *Pediatr*, **31**, 786–801.

Thiessen H, Jacobsen J & Brodersen R (1972) Displacement of albumin-bound bilirubin by fatty acids. *Acta Paediat Scand*,**61**, 285–288.

Winick M & Rosso P (1969) The effect of severe early malnutrition on cellular growth of human brain. *Pediat Res*, **3**, 181–84.

Chapter 18 · Enteral Nutrition for Infants and Children

Requirements for normal infants

Successful breast feeding fulfills the nutritional requirements of the normal infant under six months of age. Manufacturers of infant formulae have based their composition on mature human milk (see pp. 251–2) in order to provide the bottle fed infant with an appropriate balanced nutrient intake.

Fluid, energy and protein requirements for infants are summarized in Table 18.1. Their mineral and vitamin requirements are detailed in Table 18.3.

Feeding the correct volume of a recommended infant formula until the age of six months, will ensure the infant's nutritional requirements are met. Once over six months of age continuation with an infant formula or substitution of cows' milk and a vitamin supplement together with the introduction of weaning solids will provide for the changing nutritional demands of the older infant.

Infants' requirements following injury or illness may increase and feeds should be modified accordingly.

ENTERAL FEEDING FOR INFANTS

Enteral feeding is required when an adequate energy and protein intake cannot be achieved by normal feeding.

Premature infants are often tube fed and their special needs are discussed by Francis (1986).

Table 18.1. Intake per kg/body weight *

Age (mths)	Fluid (ml)	Energy (kcal)	Protein (g)
0–6	150	100 kcal	1.85
6–9	150	95 kcal	1.65
9–12	150	100 kcal	1.50

* WHO (1985) *Protein and Energy Requirements.*

191

Infants require nasogastric feeding when:

1 oral feeds are refused or not completed.

2 the total volume of feed required cannot be taken at normal feed times, necessitating supplementary night feeds.

3 inefficient sucking restricts feed intake; this can occur with respiratory or cardiac disease, congenital malformations, e.g. cleft palate, or following long-term parenteral nutrition.

4 mental or physical handicap prevents development of normal feeding techniques.

Meeting infants' energy requirements

Infants under six months should be fed either breast milk or an infant formula. Mothers can express their own breast milk, store it in sterile bottles and refrigerate or freeze it until it is required by the infant. It can then be given down the nasogastric tube and if extra volume is required supplements of banked breast milk, or if unavailable, an infant formula, can be given (see pp. 251–2).

The nutritional quality of maternal and banked breast milk will vary, and nutrient losses, especially of fat, which adheres to the length of the tube, may occur when tube feeding. This must be taken into consideration when assessing the infant's energy intake and corresponding weight gain.

Supplements of energy as carbohydrate, fat or both, may be necessary to make up the energy deficit.

The introduction of a glucose polymer e.g. Caloreen 1 g (4 kcal) per 100 ml, increasing to 3 g (12 kcal) per 100 ml may be adequate. If weight gain remains poor, a fat emulsion such as Calogen (LCT) or Liquigen (MCT) can also be added up to 3 ml (13 kcal) per 100 ml, and will increase the total added energy content to 25 kcal per 100 ml. All additions should be made gradually. Added carbohydrate and fat can be adjusted according to the individual infants tolerance but the final proportion of energy from fat should not exceed that from carbohydrate. The same principles apply to the addition of energy supplements to standard infant formulae, to a maximum of 35 kcal per 100 ml.

As an alternative to adding a glucose polymer and fat emulsion,

Table 18.2. Handy measures for energy supplements

Scoop	Duocal or MCT Duocal	Maxijul Caloreen Polycal
Clear Square Scoop (SHS)	4 g	4 g
Red Polycal Scoop (Cow & Gate)	–	5 g
Pink SMA Gold Cap Scoop (Wyeth)	4 g	4 g
Red Premium Scoop (Cow & Gate)	5 g	5 g

Duocal (SHS) or MCT Duocal (SHS) provides both fat (40% of energy) and carbohydrate (60% of energy) in powder form. Gradual introduction starting at 2 g (9.4 kcal) per 100 ml to a maximum of 7 g (33 kcal) per 100 ml will provide one calorie per millilitre. Any feed with an energy value greater than one calorie per millimetre would be hyperosmolar and unlikely to be well tolerated. For handy measures of energy supplements see Table 18.2.

Fluid restriction

Fluid restriction in infants reduces nutrient intake. In congestive cardiac failure, the volume of infant formula or breast milk may be limited to 100–120 ml/kg actual body weight per day, depending on the degree of heart failure and the effectiveness of the diuretic therapy prescribed.

The energy requirements of these infants are high due to their increased cardiac and respiratory workload. The combination of reduced overall nutrient intake, and poor feeding due to breathlessness, exhaustion and vomiting, results in growth failure. Energy supplements, ideally in powder form in order to minimize any increase in volume, should be added to the feed.

Additions of energy to greater than one calorie per millilitre may be necessary but tolerance should be closely assessed.

Each infant's total nutrient intake should be calculated, as deficits may occur when the total volume of feed is restricted. A vitamin supplement, e.g. Abidec 0.3 ml per day is usually necessary, and trace mineral intake should be carefully monitored. Corrective cardiac surgery and an increased provision of nutrients usually results in accelerated growth.

Infants on long-term nasogastric feeding should have oral stimulation and gratification whilst being tube fed, either by using a dummy to maintain suckling or by giving small volumes by bottle or spoon. At around six months, when solids would normally be introduced, it is important to stimulate this developmental process, even when the nutrient contribution of the solids taken is minimal.

Methods of feeding in infants

Intubation techniques in infants are the same as adults (see Chapter 6). There are a variety of tubes available for paediatric enteral feeding (see p. 211). Most manufacturers offer a choice of length and french gauge (i.e. external circumference in millimetres) so that the most appropriate tube can be used for the size of the child. They are all either radio opaque or have a radio opaque line running the length of the tube for X-ray identification, and some have markers at specific points to enable exact positioning.

All infant formula milks will flow easily through the narrowest tubes. Premature infants are usually oro-gastrically fed to keep the airway as free as possible, so the smallest bore, i.e. 4 fg is used. Six fg or 8 fg tend to be used for term and older infants fed nasogastrically as they are most comfortable. Introducers are not used because of the dangers of oesophageal perforation.

PVC tubes are often chosen, which stiffen when chilled, making them easier to pass. They require changing every 10 days, but most active infants, even if gloved, manage to pull tubes out, so they are usually changed more frequently than this. Less active infants, requiring long-term enteral feeding, may be happier with 6 fg polyurethane tubes which are softer and therefore more comfortable. They can remain *in situ* for up to six months. The weighted types can be difficult to pass in small infants, so initially the unweighted type should be used.

All tubes should be securely attached to the cheek with hypo-allergenic tape, i.e. Micropore. Most tolerate this well, but if the skin becomes sore, the tube should be repositioned.

The nurse in charge of the ward is responsible for the insertion of feeding tubes. The methods used to assess if the tube is positioned correctly immediately following intubation are the same as for adults (see Chapter 6). Aspiration or air flow techniques are preferred to avoid frequent X-ray exposure.

Feeds can be given by bolus or continuous infusion. Infants who have not been fed for 24 hours or have been maintained on glucose electrolyte solutions should initially have quarter strength feed introduced, then half strength 12 to 24 hours later, before starting full strength feed. Once established on full strength, energy supplements can be introduced gradually as previously discussed. Small frequent bolus feeds are usually well tolerated starting hourly and progressing to two hourly after 24 to 48 hours. If bolus feeding is not tolerated, continuous infusion using accurate syringe pumps can be used. Four hourly aspiration checks should be made for gastric emptying and the correct position of the tube.

In older infants, less frequent bolus feeds are more representative of a normal feeding pattern. Those requiring large volumes who are unable to tolerate large bolus feeds may benefit from a combination of methods with smaller three hourly bolus feeds during the day and continuous infusion overnight. Higher calorie feeds are often better tolerated when given by continuous infusion.

A less concentrated feed could be fed by bolus during the day and a more concentrated feed overnight in order to achieve an adequate calorie intake. This would also allow the infant freedom during the day for normal play and developmental activities.

The dangers of fluid overload and feed inhalation are greater with continuous infusion, making bolus feeding the method of choice. Bolus feeds must never be forced down a tube, as rapid entry of feed into the stomach may result in vomiting and therefore increase the risk of feed inhalation. Detailed charts recording feed intake, method of delivery, vomiting, urine and stool output, should be kept so that feed tolerance and procedure can be accurately assessed and modified.

Infants with vomiting or gastro-oesophageal reflux should not be continuously fed but given a small hourly bolus of thickened feed progressing to two hourly and three hourly as the vomiting settles. Maintaining a sitting position after feeds may also be beneficial. Feeds can be thickened with starch, 2–4 g cornflour or arrowroot per 100 ml, or a hemicellulose thickener such as Nestergel or Carobel, 0.5–1 g per 100 ml. The latter does not add energy to the feed and may increase stool bulk. Instant Carobel is now available which thickens the feed without cooking. Bengers, a wheat base containing enzymes which predigests and thickens the feed, can be used for older infants, when gluten and sodium are not contraindicated.

It is important to integrate parents into the established feeding procedure as soon as they wish to do so, especially for those requiring long term feeding. The nurse, however, should remain responsible for checking the tube's position before feeding, even if the parents then take over the administration of the feed.

Gastrostomy feeding

Feeding via gastrostomy in infants is required following surgical correction of oesophageal atresia, stricture or tracheo-oesophageal fistula. The tube is usually wider than a nasogastric tube, allowing all types of feed to be used including pureed weaning foods from 4–6 months of age. Transition to normal feeding in these infants is often difficult so as soon as possible following surgery, oral stimulation should be encouraged even if only 5 ml water is allowed twice per day. The gastrostomy should be maintained until adequate nutrition is achieved via the oral route, and weight gain is satisfactory.

Jejunostomy feeding

Feeding jejunostomies are rarely used but occasionally necessary following small bowel resection. Often, defined formula feeds (see pp. 256–8) are used as tolerance of normal feeds is poor. In some cases collection of upper gastrointestinal secretions by aspiration, for use with feeds via the jejunostomy may help digestion and absorption.

Recommended Daily Amounts (RDA)

The Recommended daily amounts of food energy and nutrients for groups of people in the United Kingdom are specified in a report by the Committee on Medical Aspects of Food Policy (DHSS *Report on Health and Social Subjects* 15) (see Table 18.3).

The definition given of the recommended amount of a nutrient is 'the average amount of the nutrient which should be provided per head in a group of people, if the needs of practically all members of the group are to be met'.

The recommendations for nutrients incorporate safety margins and take into account the needs for growth in children, different requirements according to sex and age and different degrees of physical activity. The recommendations for food energy are equated with the estimated average requirement within a group of people and no additions are made for safety.

It must be remembered that;

1   The recommendations relate to groups of healthy people.

2   The recommendations do not cover any increased requirements arising from disease states.

3   The recommendations for any one nutrient presupposes that those for energy and all other nutrients are to be met.

4   Requirements differ from one individual to another.

5   Requirements of an individual may change, as alterations to the composition of a diet may effect the efficiency of nutrients absorption and utilization.

Therefore, the use of these recommendations in establishing the nutrient needs of patients, should be as a *guide only* and account must always be taken of the specific requirements of individual children.

ENTERAL FEEDING FOR CHILDREN

There are three main groups of paediatric patients requiring enteral nutrition.

1   The severely ill child.

2   The handicapped child.

3   The chronically ill child.

Table 18.3. Recommended daily amounts of food energy and some nutrients for population groups in the United Kingdom. (Adapted from DHSS 1985 revision and Food and Nutrition Board (USA) 1980)

	Average expected body weight Kg[c]	Fluid ml/day for a full fuid diet[c]	Energy MJ	Energy kcal	Protein g[a]	Thiamin mg[a]	Riboflavin mg[a]	Nicotinic Acid mg[a]	Vitamin B[6] mg[b]
Infants									
0–6 months		d	d	d	d	0.3	0.4	5	0.3
6–12 months		d	d	d	d	0.3	0.4	5	0.6
Boys[a]									
1	11.5	1100	5.0	1200	30	0.5	0.6	7	0.9
2	13.5	1300	5.75	1400	35	0.6	0.7	8	0.9
3–4	16.5	1500	6.5	1560	39	0.6	0.8	9	1.3
5–6	20.0	1700	7.25	1740	43	0.7	0.9	10	1.3
7–8	25.0	1800	8.25	1980	49	0.8	1.0	11	1.6
9–11	32.0	2200	9.5	2280	57	0.9	1.2	14	1.8
12–14	44.0	2300	11.0	2640	66	1.1	1.4	16	1.8
15–17	62.0	3000	12.0	2880	72	1.2	1.7	19	2.0
Girls[a]									
1	11.0	1050	4.5	1100	27	0.4	0.6	7	0.9
2	13.5	1300	5.5	1300	32	0.5	0.7	8	0.9
3–4	16.0	1450	6.25	1500	37	0.6	0.8	9	1.3
5–6	20.0	1700	7.0	1680	42	0.7	0.9	10	1.3
7–8	25.0	1800	8.0	1900	47	0.8	1.0	11	1.6
9–11	32.0	2000	8.5	2050	51	0.8	1.2	14	1.8
12–14	50.0	2200	9.0	2150	53	0.9	1.4	16	1.8
15–17	56.0	2200	9.0	2150	53	0.9	1.7	19	2.0

	Vitamin B$_{12}$ μg[b]	Vitamin C mg[e]	Vitamin A μg[d]	Vitamin D μg	Vitamin E mg[b]	Calcium mmol[d]	Iron mmol[b]	Magnesium mmol[b]	Zinc μmol[b]
Infants									
0–6 months	0.5	20	450	7.5	3	15.0	0.11	2.0	45
6–12 months	1.5	20	450	7.5	4	15.0	0.11	2.9	75
Boys[c]									
1	2.0	20	300	10	5	15.0	0.13	6.1	150
2	2.0	20	300	10	5	15.0	0.13	6.1	150
3–4	2.5	20	300	10	6	15.0	0.14	8.2	150
5–6	2.5	20	300	k	6	15.0	0.18	8.2	150
7–8	3.0	20	400	k	7	15.0	0.18	10.2	150
9–11	3.0	25	575	k	8	17.5	0.22	14.3	225
12–14	3.0	25	725	k	8	17.5	0.22	14.3	225
15–17	3.0	30	750	k	10	15.0	0.22	16.4	225
Girls[c]									
1	2.0	20	300	10	5	15.0	0.13	6.1	150
2	2.0	20	300	10	5	15.0	0.13	6.1	150
3–4	2.5	20	300	10	6	15.0	0.14	8.2	150
5–6	2.5	20	300	k	6	15.0	0.18	8.2	150
7–8	3.0	20	400	k	7	15.0	0.18	10.2	150
9–11	3.0	25	575	k	8	17.5	0.22 m	12.3	225
12–14	3.0	25	725	k	8	17.5	0.22 m	12.3	225
15–17	3.0	30	750	k	8	15.0	0.22 m	12.3	225

a DHSS 1985 revision. b Food and Nutrition Board (USA) 1980. c Francis 1986. d See table 18.1.

e Since the recommendations are average amounts, the figures for each age range represent the amounts recommended at the middle of the range. Within each age range, younger children will need less, and older children more, than the amount recommended.

k No dietary sources may be necessary for children and adults who are sufficiently exposed to sunlight, but during the winter, children and adolescents should receive 10 μg (400 i.u.) daily by supplementation. Adults with inadequate exposure to sunlight, for example those who are housebound, may also need a supplement of 10 μg daily.

m This intake may not be sufficient for 10% of girls and women with large menstrual losses.

The severely ill, catabolic child following an infective illness, trauma or surgery

Nutritional assessment of these children is difficult. The child's weight, state of hydration, together with an assessment of the degree of catabolism (see p. 11) will give a guide to nutrient and fluid needs.

Actual protein catabolism can be estimated using the formula below (Burman 1982).

With constant blood urea	—	g/24 hours urinary urea × 3.6
With rising blood urea	—	g/24 hours urinary urea × 3.6 + rise in blood urea (g/1) × 1.8 × body weight (kg).

As a guide, initial protein intake should be increased to twice the normal requirement (see Table 18.3) except in patients with severe burns or protein-losing enteropathies when requirements are much higher. Blood urea will rise if an excessive protein intake is given, so constant monitoring is essential. Energy intake should be increased by 20–30% with a further increase of 10% for each 1°C rise in body temperature (Burman 1982). Adjustments in both protein and energy may be required to maintain a positive nitrogen balance.

Fluid and electrolyte balance must be monitored and recorded accurately. Vitamin and mineral requirements will be increased so an intake above the RDA must be provided.

As the child's condition stabilizes, their requirements must be reassessed. Enteral feeding should be continued whilst energy and protein requirements remain raised. As oral feeding is reestablished, intermittent enteral feeding, between meals and overnight, is a useful means of maintaining an adequate intake until oral feeding plus nutritional supplements can maintain total nutrition.

The handicapped child unable to swallow or take adequate amounts of normal food

The nutritional requirements of these children are determined by their present nutritional status and mobility. Often they have been fed a more fluid diet as their condition deteriorates, the nutritional adequacy of which depends on the composition of the fluid diet used. Fat stores may be depleted due to an inadequate energy intake and muscle wasting, resulting from immobility, will have been accentuated by a reduced protein intake.

Initially, enteral feeding should provide a high energy and protein intake, appropriate to the patients' weight and height rather than their age, with a complete vitamin and mineral complement. This will replenish fat stores and, with physiotherapy, improve muscle tone. Once nutritional status has improved, the regimen must be adjusted to prevent excess fat deposition but allow for normal growth and maintainence.

Immobility reduces energy requirements, however, if there is uncontrolled increased muscular activity, energy requirements will be higher. Intercurrent infections will significantly increase energy requirements in all handicapped children, regardless of their mobility. Regular assessment and monitoring of individual children is essential to prevent under or over nutrition.

Long term enteral feeding is necessary when recovery of oral feeding is unable to support total nutrition. Often a combination of oral fluids, soft foods, and enteral feeds is the most appropriate way of maintaining an adequate nutritional intake whilst continuing to provide oral gratification, one of the few pleasures available to the severely handicapped child.

The chronically ill child requiring nutritional support

Anorexia is a major problem associated with chronic illness. Attempts to stimulate an appetite by the provision of small, familiar 'home cooked' favourites, tempting nibbles and snack foods, luxurious 'MacDonalds' style milk shakes etc. stretch both parents' and dietitian's imagination, but may only achieve a limited nutritional intake. Refreshing fruits and salads are often enjoyed, but unfortunately contribute few calories to the day's intake. The vicious circle of weakness and lethargy can reduce food intake to nothing. The value of short term enteral nutrition under these circumstances has not been fully investigated, and consequently, is probably, underestimated.

Patients with malignancy undergoing radiotherapy or chemotherapy tend to feel nauseated and are prone to vomiting following treatment. In those severely affected, short term parenteral nutrition can prevent weight loss which assists recovery and an improvement in appetite. In those less severely affected, enteral feeding delivered slowly as a continuous infusion, may be tolerated. This may be seen as another invasive procedure in children who have already undergone numerous procedures, but its relative safety and significantly reduced cost must not be forgotten. The volume tolerated may not be adequate for optimal rutrition, but is usually a great improvement on that achieved by normal feeding.

Supplementary enteral nutrition in patients with cystic fibrosis has, in the short term, improved nutritional status, weight gain, and growth. Elemental, and whole protein formulae with pancreatic enzyme supplements, have both been used successfully. Feeding overnight does not interfere with normal daily life and can provide the extra intake necessary to meet their increased nutritional requirements. Long term benefits are still to be assessed.

Unfortunately there are many examples where nutrition is suboptimal in chronic illness and where enteral feeding is probably not yet used to its full potential.

Enteral feeds for children

Semi-solid or liquid diets, if prepared as varied and appetizing meals and drinks, with appropriate vitamin and mineral supplementation, can provide an adequate nutritional intake in children unable to take normal food (see Chapter 6 and Francis 1986). However, it can be difficult for parents and nurses to achieve the required oral intake and so tube feeding becomes necessary to provide optimal nutrition.

Hospital-prepared tube feeds are a bacteriological hazard and require regular microbiological monitoring (Anderton *et al.* 1986). At present, there is no nutritionally complete whole protein feed specifically designed for children, but for children over one year of age, and greater than 10 kg body weight, either an adapted infant formula, the combination of an infant formula with an adult enteral feed or an adapted adult enteral feed can be used, see Table 18.4.

Modification of adult enteral feeds for children

Having established the protein requirement of the child the volume of feed needed to provide this quantity of protein can be calculated. All adult enteral feeds need additional energy and some, depending on the volume used, need vitamin and mineral supplementation.

Table 18.5 provides a guide to the feed volume required to meet the RDA for protein in different age groups and gives details of supplements that are necessary when the stated volume of feed is used. If the requirements of any nutrients are above the RDA, the volume of feed used should be increased or appropriate supplements given.

As most feeds contain one kcal per ml. any addition of energy necessitates an equal addition of fluid. A more concentrated feed is only necessary when energy requirements exceed volume tolerance.

Fluid energy supplements e.g. Liquid Duocal, Liquid Maxijule, Neutral Fortical etc. are incorporated easily into the feed and can be added by the nursing staff, when the feed is transferred to the feeding reservoir. Powdered energy supplements have to be liquidized into the feed, which can introduce a risk of bacterial contamination if equipment is not adequately sterilized, and blockage of feeding equipment is more likely if mixing is incomplete. However, powdered energy supplements are cheaper than fluid energy supplements and no wastage occurs. All these factors, as well as individual patient tolerance, must be considered when chosing which energy supplement to use.

Some of the adult enteral feeds do not quite meet the RDA for Vitamin D, magnesium and zinc for specific age groups. Therefore, when adapted and administered on a long term basis, it is

Table 18.4. An example of a feeding regime for a four year old girl requiring 37 g protein and 1500 kcal in 1500 ml using the addition of a fluid energy supplement.

	Volume	Vol. per feed	Protein (g)	kcal
Isocal	1200 ml	150 ml	38.4	1212
Liquid Maxijule	160 ml	20 ml	–	299
Sterile Water	160 ml	20 ml	–	–
Total Volume	1520 ml	190 ml	38.4	1511

Feed delivered in eight boluses of 190 ml every three hours.

important to monitor Vitamin D and trace element intake, especially magnesium and zinc.

Methods of feeding in children

Chapter 6 discusses the administration of enteral feeds in adults. For children, choice of feeding tube (see Table 18.6) method of intubation, feed delivery and use of feeding enterostomies, are based on the same criteria.

Feed introduction should also follow the same procedure as for adults. Energy and mineral supplementation will alter the osmotic load of a feed, so it is particularly important to ensure that the feed is gradually introduced; quarter, half, three-quarter and then onto full strength feed.

Viomedex are presently the only manufacturer of feed delivery equipment specifically designed for paediatric patients. They produce small volume reservoirs, i.e 500 ml and 1000 ml bottles, which attach to standard giving sets for gravity feeding or use with feeding pumps. Their carry pack allows mobile children freedom of movement from their bedside which is a boost to their moral.

Some other manufacturers are now marketing digital feeding pumps that control flow rate accurately to one millilitre. This should allow greater use of enteral feeding pumps in paediatric enteral nutrition.

Table 18.5. A guide to the volume of adult enteral feeds for use in specific age groups when compared to the RDA[a]

		1 year or > 10 kg	2–4 years	5–8 years	9–12 years
RDA Ranges					
Boys	Protein g	30	35–39	43–49	57–62
	Energy kcals	1200	1400–1560	1740–1980	2280–2400
Girls	Protein g	27	32–37	42–47	51–53
	Energy kcal	1100	1300–1500	1680–1900	2050–2150
Clinifeed ISO	Feed Volume Required	1100	1400	1700	2000
	Protein g	30.8	39.2	47.6	56.0
	Energy kcal	1100	1400	1700	2000
	Supplements Required (b)	Energy	Energy for 3 and 4 years	Energy for 7 and 8 years	Energy for boys
Clinifeed Favour	Feed Volume Required	800	1000	1300	1600
	Protein g	30.4	38.0	49.4	60.8
	Energy kcal	800	1000	1300	1600
	Supplements Required (b)	Energy and all minerals	Energy and all minerals	Energy	Energy

Table 18.5. *continued*

		1 year or > 10 kg	2–4 years	5–8 years	9–12 years
Isocal	Feed Volume Required	1000	1200	1500	1800
	Protein g	32	38.4	48.0	57.6
	Energy kcal	1010	1212	1515	1818
	Supplements Required (b)	Energy	Energy	Energy	Energy
Enteral 400	Feed Volume Required	1000	1300	1700	2000
	Protein g	29.0	37.7	49.3	58.0
	Energy kcal	1000	1300	1700	2000
	Supplements Required (b)	Energy and calcium	Energy	Energy for 7 and 8 years	Energy for boys
Standard Fortison	Feed Volume Required	750	1000	1200	1600
	Protein g	30.0	40.0	48.0	64.0
	Energy kcal	750	1000	1200	1600
	Supplements Required (b)	Energy, all Vitamins and Minerals	Energy, all Vitamins and Minerals	Energy, all Vitamins and Minerals	Energy

Nutrauxil

Feed Volume Required	500	1000	1300	1500
Protein g	30.0	38.0	49.4	57.0
Energy kcal	500	1000	1300	1500
Supplements Required (b)	Energy and all minerals	Energy and all minerals	Energy	Energy

Ensure

Feed Volume Required	500	1100	1300	1600
Protein g	29.6	40.7	48.1	59.2
Energy kcal	650	1166	1378	1696
Supplements Required (b)	Energy and calcium	Energy	Energy	Energy

Ensure Plus

Feed Volume Required	500	600	750	1000
Protein g	31.0	37.2	46.5	62.0
Energy kcal	750	900	1125	1500
Supplements Required (b)	Energy and calcium	Energy	Energy	Energy

Table 18.5. *continued*

		1 year or > 10 kg	2–4 years	5–8 years	9–12 years
High Energy Fortison	Feed Volume Required	600	800	1000	1200
	Protein g Energy kcal	30.0 900	40.0 1200	50.0 1500	60.0 1800
	Supplements Required (b)	Energy, all Vitamins and Minerals	Energy, all Vitamins and Minerals	Energy, all Vitamins and Minerals	Energy, all Vitamins and Minerals
Triosorbon	Feed Volume Required	750	1000	1200	1500
	Protein g Energy kcal	30.0 750	40.0 1000	48.0 1200	60.0 1500
	Supplements Required (b)	Energy, all Vitamins and Minerals	Energy, all Vitamins and Minerals	Energy, all Vitamins and Minerals	Energy, all Vitamins and Minerals
Nutranel	Feed Volume Required	750	1000	1200	1500
	Protein g Energy kcal	30.0 750	40.0 1000	48.0 1200	60.0 1500

		Energy, all Vitamins and Minerals	Energy, all Vitamins and Minerals	Energy, all Vitamins and Minerals	Energy, all Vitamins and Minerals
Pepdite 2 +	Feed Volume Required	NA	1500	1700	2300
	Protein g	NA	42.0	47.6	64.4
	Energy kcal	NA	1350	1530	2070
	Supplements Required (b)	NA	Energy	Energy	Energy
Elemental 028	Feed Volume Required	NA	1700	2000	2500
	Protein g	NA	34.0	40.0	50.0
	Energy kcal	NA	1360	1600	2000
	Supplements Required (b)	NA	Energy	Energy	Energy
Flexical	Feed Volume Required	NA	1600	1800	2000
	Protein g	NA	35.2	39.6	44.0
	Energy kca	NA	1600	1800	2000

Table 18.5. *continued*

	1 year or > 10 kg	2–4 years	5–8 years	9–12 years
Flexical	NA	None	None	Protein and Energy (use larger volume as tolerated)
Supplements Required (b)				

N/A Not applicable. Use appropriate infant formulae. (See appendix)

[a]see Table 18.3.

[b]The RDA for the following nutrients are not met by the volumes of feed stated. Supplements should be given when on long term feeding.

Clinifeed Iso — Magnesium.

Clinifeed Favor — Magnesium and Zinc.

Nutrauxil — Magnesium, Zinc and Nicotinic Acid.

Ensure — Magnesium.

All feeds — Vitamin D.

Fortison Standard
Fortison High Energy — Magnesium and Zinc.

Pepdite 2+ — Magnesium.

Elemental 028 — Magnesium.

Enteral 400 — Magnesium.

Table 18.6. Paediatric feeding tubes

	Material	Length cm	Gauge	Luer	Guidewire
Infants feeding	PVC	41	4 fg	Female	No
tube (Portex)	PVC	50	6/8 fg	Female	No
	PVC	60	10 fg	Female	No
Paediatric Silk tube (E. Merck)					
Weighted	Polyurethane	56	6 fg	Female	Yes
Unweighted	Polyurethane	56	6 fg	Female	Yes
X-Ray opaque Infant feeding tube. (Vygon code 310)	PVC	40	4/7 fg	Female	No
	PVC	50	8/12 fg	Female	No
Infant feeding tube for incubators (Vygon code 312)	PVC	125	4/12 fg	Female	No
Paediatric feeding tube. (Viomedex code VX554)	Polyurethane	65	8 fg	Male	No
Feeding tubes (Argyle)	Silicone	30	3.5 fg	Female	No
	Silicone	38	5/8 fg	Female	No
	Silicone	90	5 fg	Female	No
	Silicone	105	8/10 fg	Female	No

Complications

Diarrhoea can be a problem in children as well as in adults. Some of the causes are detailed in Chapter 6.

Vomiting occurs more frequently in children than in adults, especially in the younger age range, and can lead to feed inhalation. Alteration to the method of feed delivery in order to find the most suitable regimen for an individual child, may reduce the frequency of vomiting.

Monitoring

Careful recording of feed volume, method of delivery, vomiting and stool frequency allows assessment of a patient's tolerance of an enteral feed. Initially, daily weighing and analysis of actual nutritional intake ensures the nutritional adequacy of the feed can be assessed and adjustments made accordingly. Anthropometric measurements (see Chapter 1) provide useful data in patients who may be enterally fed on a long term basis. Height and weight should be plotted on a percentile chart (see Appendix) at regular intervals to enable judgement of an individual child's growth when compared to the normal range.

REFERENCES

Anderton A, Howard JP & Scott DW (1986) Microbiological control in enteral feeding. *Human Nutr: Appl Nutr*, **40A**, 163–7.

Burman D (1982) Nutrition in Early Childhood. In McLaren DS and Burman D eds. *Textbook of Paediatric Nutrition*, 2nd ed, pp 39–73 Churchill Livingstone, Edinburgh.

DHSS (1979) (revised 1985) *Recommended Daily Amounts of food Energy and Nutrients for Groups of People in the United Kingdom*. Report No **15**, HMSO London.

Francis D (1986) *Nutrition for Children*. Blackwell Scientific Publications, Oxford.

Lawson D (1984) Cystic Fibrosis Horizons. *Proceedings of the 9th International Cystic Fibrosis Congress*. John Wiley and Sons, Brighton, England.

National Research Council (1980) *Food and Nutrition Board Recommended Dietary Allowance*, 9th revised edn. National Academy of Sciences, Washington DC.

WHO (1985) Energy and Protein Requirements. Report of a Joint FAO/WHO/UNU Expert Consultation. *WHO Technical Report Series*, No **724**. WHO Geneva.

Chapter 19 · Parenteral Nutrition at Home

The rationale

Some patients need TPN for many months and a few need it indefinitely because of extensive intestinal disease or massive bowel resection. If they are otherwise well, it makes good sense to allow these patients to administer their nutrients at home. It is over 15 years since this was first done in the USA where there is an added financial incentive for patients to leave hospital as soon as is practicable. Since then many hundreds of patients around the world have been adequately maintained by self-administered TPN whilst leading normal active lives. One such British patient was nourished in this way throughout her normal pregnancy.

The term 'home parenteral nutrition' (HPN) has been adopted for this practice and a comparison is frequently drawn with home haemodialysis. There are many similarities, such as the need to master aseptic techniques, and the concept of intestinal failure is a useful one but the comparison perhaps dramatises HPN. In our limited experience and in the much greater experience of many centres in North America, most patients of reasonable confidence, intelligence and circumstances can be taught to administer their own parenteral nutrition safely. Although the procedures involved are very different, they are little more complex than those necessary to manage an ileostomy. Any patient considered for HPN must, of course, be metabolically stable on their chosen feeding regimen.

Venous access

We have used the Nutricath S (Vygon) successfully for up to six months in patients having TPN at home. However, for planned long-term feeding, a more robust catheter of the Broviac or

Hickman type is better. These catheters have a proximal Luer lock fitting and, several centimetres distal, a short encircling ring or 'cuff' of dacron. When the catheter is appropriately placed, this dacron cuff lies in the catheter's subcutaneous tunnel and becomes bound in the tissues.

Catheter placement should be carried out in an operating theatre with provision for radiological screening. General or local anaesthesia can be used. We have found the most convenient approach to be a cut down onto the cephalic vein in the delto-pectoral groove. The vein lies more deeply and laterally than is often thought. Once the vein is found, the tip of the catheter is brought through the subcutaneous tunnel from the selected skin entry site until the dacron cuff lies well within the tunnel. The catheter can then be cut to what is judged to be the correct length and fed through the cephalic and subclavian veins into the superior vena cava or right atrium. The position is then checked radiologically before the wound is closed. Two or three sutures are used to hold the hub initially but after a week or so, when the dacron cuff is firmly bound, these can be discarded.

The catheter can be used immediately for continuous infusion or, as is more common for patients at home, overnight infusion of nutrients. When not in use the catheter can be 'locked' by filling it with heparin in saline (1000 units in 5 ml) and fitting a Luer-Lock cap. The patient is taught to dress, connect and disconnect the catheter using aseptic technique and taking precautions to avoid air embolism. Once he or she is confident in this, and in the management of the nutrient infusion, arrangements can be made for the necessary equipment and nutrients to be supplied at home. A trial at home, under the guidance of a nurse trained in TPN techniques, is imperative before the patient is left to cope alone, or with the help of a relative. Catheter sepsis, although less common than might be expected, is still a frequent occurrence. When there is a purulent discharge from the skin entry site and no systemic symptoms it is acceptable to treat the infection with antibiotics after culturing both a swab from the site and blood withdrawn through the catheter. When there is any evidence of septicaemia the catheter must be removed.

Partially to overcome the problem of sepsis, a totally implantable device, the Port-a-cath (Pharmacia) has been developed. The silicone rubber catheter attaches to a subcutaneous stainless steel chamber with a self-sealing silicone septum. Infusions are given and blood can be withdrawn through the system using a specially-designed Huber point needle passed through the skin and portal septum.

Giving systems

A variety of giving systems has been used. Centres around the world devised their own before commerical systems were avilable. One prestigious unit uses a simple giving set without any flow control and even adds a pressure bag around the fluid container to increase the rate of flow and so complete the infusion of a day's feed over a few hours at night. Most centres, on the other hand, employ volumetric infusion pumps with many safety features and alarms.

A number of ingenious devices allow the patient full mobility whilst being fed intravenously. The best known of these are the Houston vest, designed by Dr Stanley Dudrick's group, which incorporates pockets to carry fluid containers and a mechanical pump, and the Montpelier collar. In general, however, if the nutrients can be infused overnight without glucose or fluid intolerance, this is the best course. It leaves the patient free of encumberances during the working day.

Nutrient supplies

In the USA specialist pharmacies have sprung up here and there to supply nutrients for HPN patients. Elsewhere, pharmaceutical firms already manufacturing nutrient solutions have instituted home delivery services. For HPN patients living close to their hospital there are many advantages to having their prescription for nutrients dispensed by the hospital pharmacy. Many days' supply can be stored at home in a domestic freezer.

United Kingdom HPN Register

A UK register of patients receiving parenteral nutrition at home was set up in 1977. The aim was to collect data on patients, their indications for and length of treatment, quality of life and complications, in order to improve case selection and techniques. In nine years 28 centres registered 200 patients of whom 90 suffered from Crohn's disease. Over half of all the patients were either in full-time employment or looking after a home and family unaided (Mughal & Irving 1986).

Doctors wishing to contribute to the register should write to:

The UK Home Parenteral Nutrition Register,

c/o The Department of Surgery,

Clinical Sciences Building,

Hope Hospital (University of Manchester School of Medicine),

Eccles Old Road,

SALFORD. M6 8HD.

REFERENCES

Mughal M & Irving M (1986) Home Parenteral Nutrition in the United Kingdom and Ireland: A report of 200 cases. *Lancet*, **ii**, 383–7.

Appendices

COMMON MEASURES AND CONVERSION FACTORS

Weight

1 Kilogram (kg)	=	2.2 pounds (lb)
1 oz	=	28.35 grams (g)
1 lb	=	453.6 g

Volume

1 litre	=	1.76 pints
1 pint	=	20 fluid oz = 568 ml

Protein 1 gram nitrogen = 6.25 grams protein

Energy 1 kilocalorie – 4.184 kilojoules
(kcal) (kJ)

Amount of substance

Conversion of grams to moles

Na mg × 0.043 = mmol	Cu mg × 0.015 = mmol
K mg × 0.025 = mmol	Zn mg × 0.015 = mmol
Cl mg × 0.028 – mmol	Cr mg × 0.019 = mmol
Fe mg × 0.018 – mmol	F mg × 0.052 = mmol
Ca mg × 0.025 = mmol	Se mg = 0.013 × mmol
P mg × 0.032 × mmol	Mo mg × 0.010 = mmol
Mg mg × 0.041 – mmol	I mg × 0.0078 = mmol
Mn mg × 0.018 = mmol	

Vitamins*

Vitamin A 1 μg = 3.33 international units IU
Vitamin D 1 μg = 40 international units IU
Vitamin E 1 mg d-α-tocopherol = 1.49 international units IU

---

*From Bieri JG & McKenna MC (1981) Expressing dietary values for fat-soluble vitamins: changes in concepts and terminology. *American Journal of Clinical Nutrition*, **34**, 289–295.

OPTIMAL WEIGHT RANGE FOR ADULTS ACCORDING TO HEIGHT AND FRAME

| Height without shoes | | | Desirable weight in kilograms and pounds (in indoor clothing), ages 25 and over | | | | | |
| | | | Small frame | | Medium frame | | Large frame | |
metres	ft	in	kg	lb	kg	lb	kg	lb
Men								
1.550	5	1	50.8–54.4	112–120	53.5–58.5	118–129	57.2–64	126–141
1.575	5	2	52.2–55.8	115–123	54.9–60.3	121–133	58.5–65.3	129–144
1.600	5	3	53.5–57.2	118–126	56.2–61.7	124–136	59.9–67.1	132–148
1.625	5	4	54.9–58.5	121–129	57.6–63	127–139	61.2–68.9	135–152
1.650	5	5	56.2–60.3	124–133	59 –64.9	130–143	62.6–70.8	138–156
1.675	5	6	58.1–62.1	128–137	60.8–66.7	134–147	64.4–73	142–161
1.700	5	7	59.9–64	132–141	62.6–68.9	138–152	66.7–75.3	147–166
1.725	5	8	61.7–65.8	136–145	64.4–70.8	142–156	68.5–77.1	151–170
1.750	5	9	63.5–68	140–150	66.2–72.6	146–160	70.3–78.9	155–174
1.775	5	10	65.3–69.9	144–154	68 –74.8	150–165	72.1–81.2	159–179
1.800	5	11	67.1–71.7	148–158	69.9–77.1	154–170	74.4–83.5	164–184
1.825	6	0	68.9–73.5	152–162	71.7–79.4	158–175	76.2–85.7	168–189
1.850	6	1	70.8–75.7	156–167	73.5–81.6	162–180	78.5–88	173–194
1.875	6	2	72.6–77.6	160–171	75.7–83.5	167–185	80.7–90.3	178–199
1.900	6	3	74.4–79.4	164–175	78.1–86.2	172–190	82.7–92.5	182–204

Women

1.425	4	8	41.7–44.5	92–98	43.5–48.5	96–107	47.2–54	104–119
1.450	4	9	42.6–45.8	94–101	44.5–49.9	98–110	48.1–55.3	106–122
1.475	4	10	43.5–47.2	96–104	45.8–51.3	101–113	49.4–56.7	109–125
1.500	4	11	44.9–48.5	99–107	47.2–52.6	104–116	50.8–58.1	112–128
1.525	5	0	46.3–49.9	102–110	48.5–54	107–119	52.2–59.4	115–131
1.550	5	1	47.6–51.3	105–113	49.9–55.3	110–122	53.5–60.8	118–134
1.575	5	2	49 –52.6	108–116	51.3–57.2	113–126	54.9–62.6	121–138
1.600	5	3	50.3–54	111–119	52.6–58	116–130	56.7–64.4	125–142
1.625	5	4	51.7–55.8	114–123	54.4–61.2	120–135	58.5–66.2	129–146
1.650	5	5	53.5–57.6	118–127	56.2–63	124–139	60.3–68	133–150
1.675	5	6	55.3–59.4	122–131	58.1–64.9	128–143	62.1–69.9	137–154
1.700	5	7	57.2–61.2	126–135	59.9–66.7	132–147	64 –71.7	141–158
1.725	5	8	59 –63.5	130–140	61.7–68.5	136–151	65.8–73.9	145–163
1.750	5	9	60.8–65.3	134–144	63.5–70.3	140–155	67.6–76.2	149–168
1.775	5	10	62.6–67.1	133–148	65.3–72.1	144–159	69.4–79	153–174

Based on weights of insured persons in the United States associated with lowest mortality (*Statist bull Metrop Life Insur Co* 40, Nov–Dec 1959).

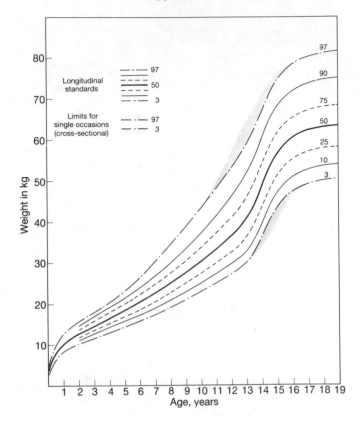

**GROWTH AND DEVELOPMENT CHARTS
(AFTER TANNER & WHITEHOUSE 1976)**

BOYS' WEIGHT

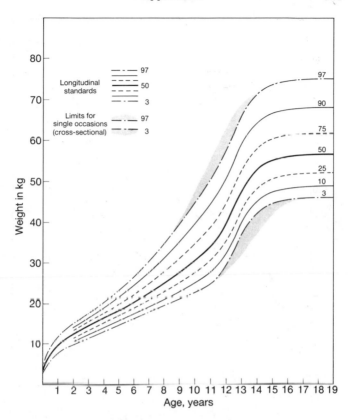

GIRLS' WEIGHT

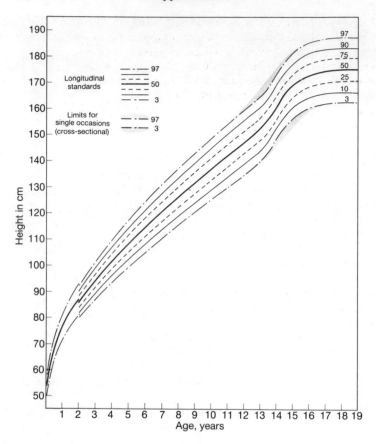

Longitudinal standards
— · — 97
——— 50
- - - 3

Limits for single occasions (cross-sectional)
— · · — 97
— · — 3

BOYS' HEIGHT

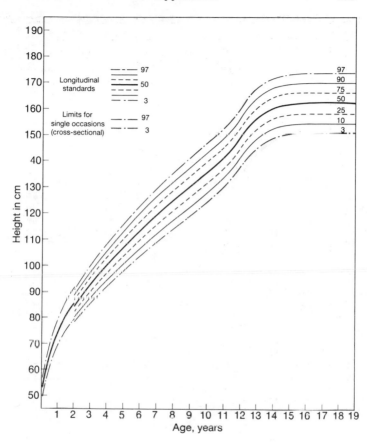

GIRLS' HEIGHT

STANDARD BASAL METABOLIC RATES
FOR INDIVIDUALS OF BOTH SEXES*

(1 MJ = 239 kcal)

Body weight (kg)	MJ/24 h m	f	Body weight (kg)	MJ/24 h m	f	Body weight (kg)	MJ/24 h m	f
3	0.5	0.6	31	5.0	4.6	59	6.7	5.6
4	0.8	0.8	32	5.0	4.6	60	6.8	5.6
5	1.0	1.0	33	5.1	4.7	61	6.8	5.7
6	1.2	1.3	34	5.2	4.7	62	6.9	5.7
7	1.5	1.6	35	5.2	4.8	63	7.0	5.8
8	1.8	1.8	36	5.3	4.8	64	7.0	5.8
9	2.0	2.1	37	5.4	4.8	65	7.0	5.9
10	2.3	2.3	38	5.5	4.9	66	7.1	5.9
11	2.6	2.6	39	5.5	4.9	67	7.1	6.0
12	2.8	2.8	40	5.6	4.9	68	7.2	6.0
13	3.0	3.0	41	5.6	5.0	69	7.2	6.0
14	3.2	3.2	42	5.7	5.0	70	7.3	6.1
15	3.4	3.4	43	5.8	5.0	71	7.3	6.1
16	3.6	3.5	44	5.8	5.1	72	7.3	6.1
17	3.7	3.6	45	5.9	5.1	73	7.4	6.2
18	3.8	3.7	46	6.0	5.1	74	7.4	6.2
19	3.9	3.8	47	6.0	5.2	75	7.5	6.2
20	4.0	3.9	48	6.1	5.2	76	7.5	6.3
21	4.1	3.9	49	6.1	5.2	77	7.6	6.3
22	4.2	4.0	50	6.2	5.3	78	7.6	6.3
23	4.3	4.0	51	6.3	5.3	79	7.7	6.4
24	4.4	4.1	52	6.3	5.3	80	7.7	6.4
25	4.5	4.2	53	6.4	5.4	81	7.7	6.5
26	4.6	4.2	54	6.4	5.4	82	7.8	6.5
27	4.7	4.3	55	6.5	5.4	83	7.8	6.6
28	4.7	4.4	56	6.6	5.5	84	7.8	6.6
29	4.8	4.5	57	6.6	5.5	85	7.9	6.6
30	4.9	4.5	58	6.7	5.5			

Not applicable to the elderly.

For men over 60 years use $BMR = 0.049 (wt) + 2.46$, or $BMR = 0.038 (wt) + 4.07 (ht) - 3.49$.

For women over 60 years use $BMR = 0.038 (wt) + 2.76$, or $BMR = 0.033 (wt) + 1.92 (ht) + 0.07$.

*Schofield W.N., Schofield Claire and James W.P.T., (1985) Basal metabolic rate—Review and prediction, together with an annotated bibliography of source material. Supplement to Human Nutrition: Clinical Nutrition Vol 39C Suppl. 1 p 1–96.

CONSTITUENTS OF LIPID INFUSION SOLUTIONS

Travamulsion (Travenol)

	Travamulsion 10%	Travamulsion 20%
Per litre		
Soya bean oil (g)	100	200
Egg phosphatide (g)	12	12
Glycerin (g)	22.5	22.5
Energy approx (kcal)	1100	2000

Sodium Hydroxide is added for pH adjustment

Intralipid (KabiVitrum)

	Intralipid 10%	Intralipid 20%
Per litre		
Soya bean oil (g)	100	200
Egg phospholipid (g)	12	12
Glycerol (g)	22.5	22.5
Phosphate (mmol)	15	15
Energy (kcal)	1100	2000
Fatty acid content	Linoleic acid 55% Palmitic acid 8.5% Linolenic acid 8% Stearic acid 8% Oleic acid 25% Other fatty acids 0.5%	
Vitamin E	Variable content depending on the soya crop Average figure: 500 ml 20% Intralipid ≡ 20 mg d-α-tocopherol	

Lipofundin S (B Braun)*

	Lipofundin S 10%	Lipofundin S 20%
Per litre		
Soya bean oil (g)	100	200
Soya bean lecithin (g)	7.5	15
Glycerol (g)	25	25
Energy (kcal)	1068	2035

CONSTITUENTS OF LIPID INFUSION SOLUTIONS *(continued)*

Lipofundin MCT/LCT (B Braun)*

Per litre	Lipofundin MCT/LCT 10%	Lipofundin MCT/LCT 20%
Soya bean oil (g)	50	100
Medium chain triglycerides (g)	50	100
Egg lecithin (g)	12	12
Glycerol (g)	25	25
Energy (kcal)	1058	1910

*These products are awaiting DHSS approval but are available on a named patient basis.

AMINO ACID CONTENT OF COMMERCIALLY AVAILABLE SOLUTIONS

L—amino-acids g/10 g Nitrogen	Aminofusin 1600, L 1000, L Forte (Merck)	Aminoplasmal L3, L5, L10 (Braun)	Aminoplasmal Ped (Braun)	Aminoplex 5, and 12 (Geistlich)	Aminoplex 14, (Geistlich)	Aminoplex 24 (Geistlich)	Freamine (Boots)	Perifusin (Merck)	Synthamin 9, 14 + 17 (Travenol)	Travenol branched chain amino-acid (4%)	Vamin 9 + Vamin 9 glucose (KabiVitrum)	Vamin 14 + 18 (KabiVitrum)	Nephramine (Boots)
N—acetyl-L-tyrosine	—	0.77	1.16	—	—	—	—	—	—	—	—	—	—
L—alanine	7.89	8.53	7.84	8.36	11.0	8.3	4.28	7.92	12.4	—	3.3	8.7	—
L—arginine	5.26	5.73	2.97	7.4	6.8	7.67	2.2	5.28	7.0	—	3.6	6.2	—
L—aspargine	—	2.32	1.23	—	—	—	—	—	—	—	—	—	—
L—aspartic acid	—	0.81	2.57	—	—	—	—	—	—	—	4.5	1.8	—
L—cysteine	—	0.45	1.97	—	—	—	—	—	—	—	1.6	0.3	—
L—glutamic acid	11.84	2.86	13.24	1.6	—	1.67	—	11.88	—	—	1	3	—
Glycine (aminoacetic acid)	13.16	4.92	6.62	3.54	8.35	3.67	12.1	13.2	—	—	2.3	4.3	—
L—histidine	1.32	3.24	4.05	1.28	2.05	1.83	1.7	1.32	6.2	—	2.7	3.8	2.8
L—isoleucine	2.04	3.18	1.89	3.36	2.35	3.17	4.21	2.12	2.9	23	4.3	3	6.2
L—leucine	2.89	5.54	3.58	4.36	3.28	4.83	5.5	2.9	3.6	23	5.9	4.3	9.8
L—lysine	3.29	4.36	6.08	5.48	6.34	4.53	6.21	3.3	4.4	—	4.3	4.9	10
L—methionine	2.76	2.37	1.08	3.66	4.78	4	3.21	2.78	3.5	—	2.1	3	9.8
L—ornithine	—	1.99	1.54	1.6	1.49	1.67	—	—	2.4	—	—	—	—
L—phenylalanine	2.89	3.18	2.56	5.64	3.28	5.73	3.42	2.9	3.4	—	6.1	4.3	9.8
L—proline	9.21	5.54	3.65	9.66	2.99	10	6.78	9.24	4.1	—	9	3.8	—
L—serine	—	1.49	1.35	1.94	—	2	3.57	—	3	—	8.3	2.5	—
L—threonine	1.32	2.55	4.05	2.58	2.38	2.37	2.42	1.32	2.55	—	3.3	3	4.4
L—tryptophan	0.59	1.12	0.81	1.2	1.19	1.17	0.92	0.66	1.1	—	1.1	1	2.2
L—tyrosine	—	0.19	0.41	—	—	—	—	—	0.24	—	0.6	0.12	—
L—valine	1.97	2.99	2.16	3.6	3.88	3.73	4	1.98	3.5	20.6	4.8	4	7.1

CONSTITUENTS OF AMINO ACID INFUSION SOLUTIONS (BRITISH NATIONAL FORMULARY 1986)

Preparation	Manufacturer	Nitrogen g/litre	Energy kJ/litre	Electrolytes mmol/litre					Other components/litre
				K^+	Mg^{2+}	Na^+	$Acet^-$	Cl^-	
Aminofusin L600	Merck	7.6	2500	30	5	40	10	14	sorbitol 100 g, vitamins
Aminofusin L1000	Merck	7.6	4200	30	5	40	10	14	ethanol 5.28%, sorbitol 100 g, vitamins
Aminofusin L Forte	Merck	15.2	1700	30	5	40	10	27.5	vitamins
Aminoplasmal L3	Braun	4.82	510	25	2.5	48	59	18	$H_2PO_4^-$ 9 mmol, malate 7.5 mmol
Aminoplasmal L5	Braun	8.03	850	25	2.5	48	59	31	$H_2PO_4^-$ 9 mmol, malate 7.5 mmol
Aminoplasmal L10	Braun	16.06	1700	25	2.5	48	59	62	$H_2PO_4^-$ 9 mmol, malate 7.5 mmol
Aminoplasmal Ped	Braun	7.4	850	25	2.5	50	27	15	
Aminoplex 5	Geistlich	5.0	4200	28	4	35	28	43	ethanol 5%, sorbitol 125 g, malic acid 1.85 g
Aminoplex 12	Geistlich	12.44	1300	30	2.5	35	5	67	malic acid 4.6 g
Aminoplex 14	Geistlich	13.4	1400	30		35		79	vitamins, malic acid 5.36 g
Aminoplex 24	Geistlich	24.9	2600	30	2.5	35	5	67	malic acid 4.5 g
FreAmine III 8.5%	Boots	13.0	1400			10	72	<3	HPO_4^{2-} 10 mmol
FreAmine III 10% pH 6.5	Boots	15.3	1650			10	88	<2	HPO_4^{2-} 10 mmol

Glucoplex 1000	Geistlich		4200	30	2.5	50		67	$H_2PO_4^-$ 18 mmol, Zn^{2+} 0.046 mmol, anhydrous glucose 240 g
Glucoplex 1600	Geistlich		6700	30	2.5	50		67	$H_2PO_4^-$ 18 mmol, Zn^{2+} 0.046 mmol, anhydrous glucose 400 g
Nephramine	Boots	6.5	700	30		5	44		essential amino acids only
Perifusin	Merck	5.0	550	30	5	40	10		malate 22.5 mmol
Synthamin 9	Travenol	9.1	1000	60	5	73	100	70	$H_2PO_4^-$ 30 mmol
Synthamin 14	Travenol	14.0	1600	60	5	73	130	70	$H_2PO_4^-$ 30 mmol
Synthamin 14 without electrolytes	Travenol	14.0	1600				68	34	
Synthamin 17	Travenol	16.5	1900	60	5	73	150	70	$H_2PO_4^-$ 30 mmol
Branched chain amino acid solution	Travenol	4.4	500						
Vamin 9	KabiVitrum	9.4	1000	20	1.5	50		55	Ca^{2+} 2.5 mmol
Vamin 9 glucose	KabiVitrum	9.4	2700	20	1.5	50		55	Ca^{2+} 2.5 mmol, anhydrous glucose 100 g
Vamin 14	KabiVitrum	13.5	1400	50	8	100	135	100	Ca^{2+} 5 mmol, SO_4^{2-} 8 mmol
Vamin 14 (electrolyte-free)	KabiVitrum	13.5	1400						
Vamin 18 (electrolyte-free)	KabiVitrum	18.0	1900						

ELECTROLYTE SOURCE SOLUTIONS

Ion	Source solution	Example of commercial source	Ion content (mmol/ml)
Ca^{++}	Calcium Chloride		
	$(CaCl_2 2H_2O)$ 13.4%	Evans	0.9
	Calcium gluconate		
	$(C_{12}H_{22}CaO_{14}H_2O)$ 10%	Evans	0.22
K^+	Addiphos	KabiVitrum	1.5
	Potassium Acetate		
	(CH_3COOK) 49%	Not available*	5.0
	Potassium chloride (KCl) 15%	Macarthy	2.0
	Potassium chloride (KCl) 20%	Macarthy	2.7
	Potassium phosphate		
	(K_2HPO_4) 17.4%	Macarthy	2.0
Mg^{++}	Magnesium sulphate		
	$(MgSO_4 7H_2O)$ 50%	Evans	2.0
Na^+	Addiphos	KabiVitrum	1.5
	Sodium aceate		
	$(CH_3COONa\ 3H_2O)$ 34.1%	Not available*	2.5
	Sodium bicarbonate		
	$(NaHCO_3)$ 8.4%	Macarthy	1.0
	Sodium chloride (NaCl) 30%	Macarthy	5.0
	Sodium phosphate		
	$(Na_2HPO_4\ 12H_2O)$ 26.9%	Not available*	1.5
Cl^-	Potassium chloride (KCl) 15%	Macarthy	2.0
Phosphate	Addiphos	KabiVitrum	2.0
	Potassium phosphate		
	(K_2HPO_4) 17.4%	Macarthy	1.0
	Sodium phosphate		
	$(Na_2HPO_4\ 12H_2O)$ 26.9%	Not available*	0.75
Zn^{++}	Zinc acetate		
	$(Zn(CH_3COO)_2 2H_2O)$	Not available*	0.04

* Not available commercially but prepared by the Hospital Pharmacy Department.

Carbohydrate solutions containing electrolytes

Source solution	Commercial source	Ion	Content (mmol/l)
Nutracel 400 in 20% dextrose	Travenol	Ca^{++}	15
		Cl^-	66
		Mg^{++}	18
		Mn^{++}	0.08
		Zn^{++}	0.08
Nutracel 800 in 20% dextrose	Travenol	Ca^{++}	7.5
		Cl^-	33
		Mg^{++}	9
		Mn^{++}	0.04
		Zn^{++}	0.04
Glucoplex 1000 in 24% dextrose 1600 in 40% dextrose	Geistlich	Na^+	50
		K^+	30
		Mg^{++}	2.5
		Zn^{++}	0.045
		PO_4	18
		Cl^-	67

CONTENTS OF MULTIVITAMIN SOLUTIONS FOR INTRAVENOUS USE

	Thiamin (B_1) mg	Riboflavin (B_2) mg	Pyridoxine (B_6) mg	Cyanocobalamin (B_{12}) µg	Nicotinamide mg	Biotin µg	Pantothenic acid/dexpanthenol mg	Folic acid mg	Ascorbic acid (C) mg	Calciferol (D) µg	Phytomenadione (K) µg	Retinol (A) µg	Tocopherol (E) mg
Recommended intake/day (adult) (see Chapter 1)	3.0	3.6	4.0	5	40	60	15	0.4	100	5	150	1000	10
Multibionta (10 ml) (Merck)	50	10	15	–	100	–	25	–	500	–	–	3000	5
Multiple vitamin solution (IMS) (10 ml)	50	10	15		100		25		500	25		3000	3.3
Parentrovite i.v. (Bencard) Amp 1 (5 ml)	250	4.0	50	–	–	–	–	–	–	–	–	–	–
Amp 2 (5 ml)	–	–	–	–	160	–	–	–	500	–	–	–	–
Solivito (KabiVitrum) (1 vial)	.12	1.8	2.0	2.0	10	0.3	10	0.2	30	–	–	–	–
Vitlipid adult (KabiVitrum) (10 ml)	–								–	3	150	750	–
Vitlipid infant (KabiVitrum) (1 ml)										2.5	50	100	–
Solivito N (KabiVitrum) (1 vial)	3.0	3.6	4.0	5.0	40	60	15	0.4	100				
Vitlipid N adult (KabiVitrum) (10 ml)										5	150	1000	9.1
Vitlipid N Infant (KabiVitrum) (1 ml)										1.0	20	69	0.64 µg

* (IMS) International Medication Systems (U.K.) Ltd.

INTRAVENOUS MULTIVITAMIN PREPARATIONS RECOMMENDED FOR PAEDIATRIC USE

Solution		Solivito†		MVI*		Vitlipid infant**	
		vial	dose/kg 1/10 vial	dose/kg 2 ml	vial	1 ml	4 ml
Thiamine (B1)	mg	1.2	0.12	10.0	50		
Riboflavin (B2)	mg	1.8	0.18	2.0	10		
Nicotinamide	mg	10.0	1.0	20.0	100		
Pyridoxine (B6)	mg	2.0	0.2	3.0	15		
Pantothenic acid	mg	10.0	1.0	5.0	25		
Biotin	mg	0.3	0.03				
Folic acid	mg	0.2	0.02				
Cyanocobalamin (B12)	μg	2.0	0.2				
Ascorbic acid	mg	30.0	3.0	100	500		
Retinol (A)	μg			600	3000	100	400
Calciferol (D)	μg			5	25	2.5	10
Phytomenadione (K)	μg			−	−	50	200
Tocopherol (E)	mg			0.7	3.3	−	−

†   Solivito (KabiVitrum) dose 1/10 vial/kg to max of 1 vial

*   MVI (International Medications Ltd) dose 2 mg/kg

**   Vitlipid Infant (KabiVitrum) dose 1 ml/kg to max of 4 ml

TRACE ELEMENT PREPARATIONS FOR INTRAVENOUS USE

Additrace (KabiVitrum)
One vial (10 ml) contains:

Fe^{+++}	20 μmol	F^-	50 μmol
Zn^{++}	100 μmol	Cr^{++}	0.2 μmol
Cu^{++}	20 μmol	Se^{++}	0.4 μmol
I^-	1 μmol	Mo^{++}	0.2 μmol
Mn^{++}	5 μmol		

Addamel (KabiVitrum)
One vial (10 ml) contains:

Ca^{++}	5 mmol	Cu^{++}	5 μmol
Mg^{++}	1.5 mmol	F^-	50 μmol
Fe^{+++}	50 μmol	I^-	1 μmol
Zn^{++}	20 μmol	Cl^-	13.3 μmol
Mn^{++}	40 μmol		

MTE-4 (Travenol)
One vial (10 ml) contains:

Cr^{++}	0.77 μmol	Mn^{++}	0.02 mmol
Cu^{++}	0.06 mmol	Zn^{++}	0.15 mmol

Ped-el (KabiVitrum)
contains per ml:

Ca^{++}	0.15 mmol	Cu^{++}	0.075 μmol
Mg^{++}	25 μmol	F^-	0.75 μmol
Fe^{+++}	0.5 μmol	I^-	0.01 μmol
Zn^{++}	0.15 μmol	PO_4^{---}	75 μmol
Mn^{++}	0.25 μmol	Cl^-	0.35 mmol

1 vial (20 ml) of Ped-el contains less than 1 μmol K^+ and less than 1.5 mmol Na^+

Other single source solutions

Trace element	Source solution	Manufacturer
Co^{++}	Hydroxocobalamin injection	Glaxo
Cr^{+++}	Potassium dichromate injection	Hospital pharmacy
Cu^{++}	Copper sulphate or chloride injection	Hospital pharmacy
F^-	Sodium fluoride injection	Hospital pharmacy
I^-	Potassium iodide injection	Hospital pharmacy
Mn^{++}	Manganous chloride injection	Hospital pharmacy
Se^{++}	Seleno-methionine injection	Hospital pharmacy
Zn^{++}	Zinc acetate injection	Hospital pharmacy

NB Addamel is not satisfactorily compatible with 'Synthamin' (Travenol) preparations.

COMPARISON OF INTRAVENOUS TRACE
ELEMENT SOLUTIONS FOR PAEDIATRIC USE

Solution	(units)	Addamel 1 ml	Addamel[+] (0.5 ml) dose/kg/day	Pedel[*] (4 ml) dose/kg/day	Pedel 1 ml
Calcium	(mmol)	0.5	0.25	0.6	0.15
Magnesium	(mmol)	0.15	0.075	0.1	0.025
Iron	(μmol)	5.0	2.5	2.0	0.5
Zinc	(μmol)	2.0	1.0	0.6	0.15
Manganese	(μmol)	4.0	2.0	1.0	0.25
Copper	(μmol)	0.5	0.25	0.3	0.075
Fluoride	(μmol)	5.0	2.5	0.3	0.075
Iodine	(μmol)	0.1	0.05	0.04	0.01
Phosphate	(mmol)	–	–	0.3	0.075
Chloride	(mmol)	1.33	0.66	1.4	0.35
Sorbitol	(mg)	300	150	1200	300

[+] Addamel (KabiVitrum) 0.25–0.5 ml/kg/day to max of 10 ml

[*] Pedel (KabiVitrum) 3–4 ml/kg/day to max of 30 ml

ORAL VITAMIN AND MINERAL SUPPLEMENTS

Abidec Drops (Parke Davies)
Per 0.6 ml

Vitamin A	1200	μg
Calciferol	10	μg
Thiamin hydrochloride	1	mg
Riboflavin	0.4	mg
Pyridoxine hydrochloride	0.5	mg
Nicotinamide	5	mg
Ascorbic acid	50	mg

Adults 0.6 ml daily, children up to 1 year 0.3 ml daily

Dalivit Drops (Paines & Byrne)
Per 0.6 ml

Vitamin A	1500	μg
Ergocalciferol	10	μg
Thiamin	1	mg
Riboflavin	0.4	mg
Pyridoxine	0.5	mg
Ascorbic acid	50	mg
Nicotinamide	5	mg

Children up to 1 yr 0.3 ml (7 drops)
over 1 yr 0.6 ml (14 drops)

Ketovite Tablets (Paines & Byrne)
Per tablet

Acetomenaphthone	0.5	mg
Thiamin hydrochloride	1	mg
Riboflavin	1	mg
Pyridoxine hydrochloride	0.33	mg
Nicotinamide	3.3	mg
Calcium pantothenate	1.16	mg
Ascorbic acid	16.6	mg
Tocopheryl acetate	5	mg
Inositol	50	mg
Biotin	0.17	mg
Folic acid	0.25	mg

Ketovite Liquid (Paines & Byrne)
Sugar free supplement per 5 ml

Vitamin A	750	μg
Vitamin D	10	μg
Choline chloride	150	mg
Cyanocobalamin	12.5	μg

Adults and children 1 tablet three times daily plus 5 ml liquid

Metabolic Mineral Mix (Scientific Hospital Supplies)

Elements	per 100 g
Sodium g	3.96
mmol	172.2
Potassium g	8.3
mmol	212.3
Chloride g	1.8
mmol	50.8
Calcium g	8.2
mmol	204.6
Phosphorous g	5.96
mmol	192.4
Magnesium g	0.97
mmol	39.9

Trace Elements	Per 100 g
Iron mg	63.0
Zinc mg	48.0
Iodine mg	0.76
Manganese mg	5.7
Copper mg	13.0
Molybdenum μg	150.0

The recommended daily intake of Metabolic Mineral Mix is 1.5 g/kg body weight for infants up to 5.5 kg. Above this weight 8 g/day is given.

Seravit (Scientific Hospital Supplies)

Typical Composition	Seravit* Per 100 g	Infant seravit Per 100 g
Magnesium mg	1250.0	625.0
Iron mg	83.2	103.1
Zinc mg	83.2	72.2
Iodine mg	0.67	0.75
Manganese mg	12.4	7.25
Copper mg	8.2	7.5
Molybdenum μg	666.0	468.5
Chromium μg	90.0	281.0
Phosphorus mg	1600.0	3000.0
Calcium mg	—	4500.0
Selenium mg	—	281.0

ORAL VITAMIN AND MINERAL SUPPLEMENTS
continued

Seravit (Scientific Hospital Supplies) *continued*

Vitamins	Per 100 g	
Vitamin A mg	6.5	6.5
Vitamin E mg	166.0	166.0
Vitamin C mg	566.0	566.0
Thiamin mg	11.6	11.6
Riboflavin mg	11.6	11.6
Pyridoxine mg	15.0	15.0
Nicotinamide mg	83.2	83.2
Pantothenic Acid mg	36.64	40.0
Meso Inositol mg	184.0	184.0
Choline μg	1832.0	1832.0
Vitamin D_3 μg	38.0	75.0
Vitamin B_{12} μg	36.0	36.0
Folic Acid μg	1660.0	1660.0
Biotin μg	1160.0	1160.0
Vitamin K_1 μg	3920.0	2000.0
Carbohydrate g	88.5	74.2
Normal daily dose	5 g/400 Kcal	8–12 g

*The seravit listed was designed for 'home made' tube feeds and does not contain Ca, Na, K. An alternative mix containing these elements is available on request from SHS.

COMPLETE NASOGASTRIC FEEDS: COMPOSITION PER LITRE FULL STRENGTH FEED

	Fortison (Cow and Gate)			
	Standard	Energy-Plus	Low Sodium	Soya
kcal	1000	1500	1000	1000
Non N kcal: Ng	131:1	167:1	131:1	131:1
Protein g (Ng)	40 (6.4)	50 (8)	40 (6.4)	40 (6.4)
Source	Sodium, calcium caseinate	Sodium, calcium caseinate	Calcium, potassium caseinate	Soya protein isolate
Fat g	40	65	40	40
Source	Corn, palm, coconut oil	Corn, palm, coconut oil	Corn, palm, coconut oil	Corn, palm coconut oil
CHO g	120	179	120	120
Source	Maltodextrin	Maltodextrin	Maltodextrin	Maltodextrin
Lactose fraction g	< 0.25	< 0.25	< 0.25	< 0.05
Na mmol	35	35	⩽ 11	36
K mmol	38	38	38	38
Cl mmol	22	22	7	22
Fe mmol	0.18	0.18	0.18	0.18
Ca mmol	12	12	12	12
P mmol	16	16	16	16
Mg mmol	6	6	6	6
Mn μmol	70	70	70	70
Cu μmol	15	15	15	15
Zn μmol	105	105	105	105
I μmol	0.5	0.5	0.5	0.5
Volume of feed to provide recommended vitamin intake	2 litres	2 litres	2 litres	2 litres
Osmotic load manufacturers figures	260 mOsm/l	320 mOsm/l	220 mOsm/l	260 mOsm/l
Preparation of full strength feed	Liquid 500 ml bottle no dilution	Liquid 500 ml bottle no dilution	Liquid 500 ml bottle no dilution	Liquid 500 ml bottle no dilution

COMPLETE NASOGASTRIC FEEDS *continued*

	Clinifeed (Roussel)			
	ISO	Favour	400	Protein Rich
kcal	1000	1000	800	1000
Non N kcal: Ng	200:1	145:1	142:1	79:1
Protein g (Ng) Source	28 (4.5) Dried skimmed milk Whey proteins	38 (6) Sodium caseinate Soya protein isolate	30 (4.8) Dried skimmed milk Whey proteins Egg yolk Potassium caseinate	60 (9.6) Whey proteins Sodium caseinate Dried skimmed milk
Fat g Source	41 Vegetable oil Butter fat	33 Maize oil MCT oil Soya oil	27 Maize oil Soya oil	22 Soya oil
CHO g Source	130 Maltodextrin	140 Maltodextrin glucose	110 Maltodextrin sucrose	140 Maltodextrin sucrose
Lactose fraction g	19	none	19	14
Na mmol	15	30	14	25
K mmol	38	28	25	43
Cl mmol	29	32	14	26
Fe mmol	0.12	0.14	0.05	0.13
Ca mmol	15	12	15	6
P mmol	14	11	17	18
Mg mmol	5	8	4	4
Mn μmol	4	36	3	54
Cu μmol	15	15	6	8
Zn μmol	135	120	90	112
I μmol	—	—	—	—
Volume of feed to provide recommended vitamin intake	2 litres long term feeding then add folate	2 litres	2.5 litres	2 litres long term feeding then add B_{12} & Biotin
Osmotic load manufacturers figures	270 mOsm/l	335 mOsm/l	255 mOsm/l	399 mOsm/l
Preparation of full strength feed	Liquid 375 ml per can no dilution	Liquid 375 ml per can no dilution	Liquid 375 ml per can +125 ml water	Liquid 375 ml per can + 125 ml water

...sure (Abbott)	Ensure Plus (Abbott)	Osmolite (Abbott)	Enrich (Abbott)	Two Cal. HN (Abbott)
...000	1500	1000	1040	2000
...53:1	125:1	126:1	148:1	125:1
35 (5.6)	62 (9.9)	42 (6.7)	38 (6)	83 (13.3)
...odium, calcium caseinate Soya protein ...olate	Sodium, calcium caseinate Soya protein isolate	Caseinates Soya protein isolate	Caseinates Soya protein isolate	Caseinates
...35	50	35	35	91
...orn oil	Corn oil	MCT Corn oil Soya oil	Corn oil	Corn oil Coconut oil
...37	200	134	153	217
...ydrolysed corn starch ...ucrose	Hydrolysed corn starch sucrose	Hydrolysed corn starch	Corn syrup solids sucrose Soya polysaccharide (11 g dietary fibre)	Corn syrup solids sucrose
...one	none	none	none	none
35	51	38	35	46
38	47	38	38	59
38	45	38	38	44
0.16	0.34	0.23	0.21	0.34
12	27	18	17	26
16	34	23	22	34
8	17	12	11	17
45	95	64	54	108
15	31	21	21	30
...69	360	243	225	360
0.6	1.2	0.8	0.0	1.2
2 litres	2 litres	2 litres	2 litres	1 litre
380 mOsm/l	500 mOsm/l	263 mOsm/l	400 mOsm/l	533 mOsm/l
Liquid 250 ml per can no dilution	Liquid 250 ml per can no dilution	Liquid 250 ml per can no dilution	Liquid 250 ml per can no dilution	Liquid 237 ml per can no dilution

COMPLETE NASOGASTRIC FEEDS *continued*

	Pulmocare (Abbott)	Isocal (Bristol-Myers)	Nutrauxil (KabiVitrum)	Liquisorb (Merck)	Enteral 400 (SHS)*
kcal	1500	980	1000	1000	1000
Non N kcal: Ng	125:1	174:1	140:1	130:1	193:1
Protein g (Ng) Source	62 (10) Sodium and calcium caseinate	32 (5) Soya protein isolate caseinate solids	38 (6) Sodium, calcium caseinate soya protein isolate	40 (6.4) Lactroproteins	29 (4.6) Whey protein isolate
Fat g Source	92 Corn oil	42 Soya oil 80% MCT oil 20%	34 Sunflower oil MCT oil 13%	40 Soya bean oil	39 Arachis oil MCT oil 25%
CHO g Source	105 Corn syrup solids	126 Glucose syrup solids	138 Oligo & poly saccharide	118 Mono, di oligo and polysaccharide	144 Maltodextrin
Lactose fraction g	none	none	< 0.1	trace	low
Na mmol	57	21	33	45	27
K mmol	49	32	32	45	30
Cl mmol	48	28	≤ 33	50	23
Fe mmol	0.34	0.16	0.18	0.13	0.18
Ca mmol	26	15	12	16	12
P mmol	34	16	19	17	16
Mg mmol	17	8	5	8	6
Mn μmol	36	55	27	22	28
Cu μmol	30	16	15	19	15
Zn μmol	360	153	112	90	156
I μmol	1.2	0.6	0.6	0.4	0.6
Volume of feed to provide recommended vitamin intake	1 litre	2 litres	2 litres	2 litres	2 litres
Osmotic load manufacurers figures	385 mOsm/l	300 mOsm/kg	350 mOsm/l	270 mOsm/l	330 mOsm/l
Preparation of full strength feed no dilution	Liquid 237 ml per can no dilution	Liquid 250 ml per can no dilution	Liquid 500 ml bottle no dilution	Liquid 4 flavours 500 ml bottle no dilution	100 g powder + 330 ml water

*Scientific Hospital Supplies

esubin Liquid resenius)	Fresubin plus F (Fresenius)	Nutricomp F (B. Braun)	Triosorbon (Merck)	HiperNutril MCT (Oxford Nut.)
000	1000	1250	1000	1000
40:1	140:1	120:1	129:1	105:1
38 (6) ilk and ya protein	38 (6) Milk protein Vegetable protein	54 (8.6) Milk protein Soya protein	40 (6.4) Whey casein	48 (7.7) Sodium caseinate lactalbumin L-cystine
34 unflower oil	34 Sunflower oil	33 Sunflower oil MCT oil	40 MCT oil 78% Sunflower oil 22%	31 MCT oil 75% EFA
38 igo and lysaccharide	138 Oligo and polysaccharide 10 g Dietary fibre	186 Maltodextrin Maltose	119 Mono, oligo, & polysaccharide Maltodextrin	124 Polysaccharides disaccharides
0 1 g	0 1 g	< 1%	trace	none
33	33	43	42	44
32	32	49	42	44
33	33	17	53	42
0.18	0.18	0.18	0.16	0.09
19	19	16	13	5
19	19	20	19	14
7	7	5	7	3
27	36	16	22	25
15	16	39	15	15
12	112	150	112	95
0.6	0.6		0.6	0.6
litres	2 litres	2 litres	2 litres	2 litres
00 mOsm/l	350 mOsm/l	340 mOsm/l	215 mOsm/l	400 mOsm/l
quid 4 flavours 00 ml bottle dilution	Liquid 2 flavours 500 ml bottle no dilution	Liquid 8 flavours 500 ml bottle no dilution	85 g sachet +400 ml water	90 g sachet + 400 ml water

COMPLETE NASOGASTRIC FEEDS *continued*

	Peptide formulae			
	Nutranel (Roussel)	Peptisorbon (Merck)	Pepdite 2+ (SHS)*	MCT Pepdite 2+ (SHS)*
kcal	1000	1000	900	920
Non N kcal: Ng	130:1	126:1	176:1	180:1
Protein g (Ng) Source	40 (6.4) Short chain peptides Free amino acids	45 (7.2) Oligopeptides 80% Amino acids 20%	28 (4.5) Hydrolysed meat and soya proteins Amino acids	28 (4.5) Hydrolysed meat and soya protein Amino acids
Fat g Source	10 MCT oil 50% Corn oil 50%	13 MCT oil 60% Sunflower oil 40%	36 Refined Vegetable oils MCT 35%	38 MCT 83% Sunflower oil
CHO g Source	187 Maltodextrin	175 Maltodextrin	126 Maltodextrin	125 Maltodextrin
Lactose fraction g	2.5	trace	none	none
Na mmol	20	60	18	27
K mmol	35	30	26	26
Cl mmol	24	40	10	10
Fe mmol	0.18	0.16	0.17	0.17
Ca mmol	11	12	10	10
P mmol	12	19	13	13
Mg mmol	4	8	6	6
Mn μmol	72	27	26	26
Cu μmol	15	15	14	14
Zn μmol	105	112	144	144
I μmol	0.5	0.6	0.6	0.6
Volume of feed to provide recommended vitamin intake	2 litres	2 litres	2 litres	2 litres
Osmotic load manufacturers figures	410 mOsm/l	400 mOsm/l	288 mOsm/kg	360 mOsm/kg
Preparation of full strength feed	101 g box +350 ml water	83 g sachet +300 ml water	100 g box +400 ml water	100 g box +400 ml water

ptide formula		Elemental formulae		
exical ristol-Myers)	Reabilan (Roussel)	Vivonex (Norwich-Eaton)	Vivonex HN (Norwich-Eaton)	Elemental 028 (SHS)*
00	1000	1000	1000	800
3:1	175:1	280:1	125:1	225:1
2 (3.5) asein drolysate nino acids % ptide 30%	31 (5) Whey and casein peptides	18 (3) Amino acids	44 (7) Amino acids	20 (3.2) Crystalline amino acids
4 ya oil 80% CT oil 20%	39 MCT Evening primrose and soya oil	1.5 Safflower oil	0.9 Safflower oil	13 Arachis oil
2 arn syrup solids apioca starch	131 Maltodextrin Starch	207 Glucose solids	211 Glucose solids	156 Maltodextrin
ane	—	none	none	none
5	27	37	33	22
2	28	30	18	24
8	52	51	52	19
0.16	0.12	0.18	0.1	0.15
4	11	13	0	9
6	14	18	11	13
8	9	9	5	5
5	27	28	17	22
5	19	17	10	12
0	124	125	75	125
0.6	0.6	0.6	0.4	0.5
litres	2 litres	2 litres	3 litres	2.5 litres
0 mOsm/kg	300 mOsm/l	550 mOsm/l	800 mOsm/l	720 mOsm/l
27 g powder water to volume 1 litre	Liquid 375 ml per can no dilution	80 g packet + water to volume of 300 ml	80 g packet + water to volume of 300 ml	100 g packet + 500 ml water

cientific Hospital Supplies

DIETARY SUPPLEMENTS

PROTEIN SUPPLEMENTS Composition per 100 g

	Skimmed milk power (Domestic)	Maxipro HBV (SHS) *	Casilan (Farley)	Forceval (Unigreg)	Protifar (Cow and Gate)	Comminuted chicken (Cow and Gate)
Major ingredients	Dried skimmed milk	Supplemented whey protein	Calcium caseinate	Calcium caseinate + Vitamins and minerals	Skimmed milk protein	Finely ground chicken meat in water
Protein g	36	88	90	55	88	7–8
Fat g	1	4	1	Tr	1.6	2.5–4
Carbohydrate g	53	Tr	Tr	30	0.5	–
Energy kcal	355	360	373	366	370	Av 60
Na mmol	24	10	4.1	5	1.3	0.4
K mmol	41	11	3	1	1.3	1.2

CARBOHYDRATE SUPPLEMENTS Composition per 100 g

Caloreen (Roussel)	Maxijul (SHS)*	Maxijul (SHS)* Per 100 ml	Polycal (Cow and Gate)	Fortical (Cow and Gate) per 100 ml	Folycose powder (Abbott)	Polycose (Abbott) per 100 ml	Hycal (Beechams) per 100 ml
Glucose polymer	Glucose polymer	Glucose polymer	Maltodextrin syrup	Maltodextrin flavouring	Glucose polymer	Glucose polymer	Flavoured liquid glucose syrup mono, di, tri and higher saccharides
–	–	–	–	–	–	–	–
–	–	–	–	–		–	–
96	96	50	94	61	94	50	01
400	375	187	380	246	380	200	248
1.8	2.0	≤1.0	2.2	0.3	4.8	3.0	0.6
0.3	0.1	≤0.1	1.3	0.2	–	–	Tr

* Scientific Hospital Supplies

DIETARY SUPPLEMENTS continued

FAT SUPPLEMENTS Composition per 100 ml

	Corn oil (Domestic)	Double Cream (Domestic)	Calogen *(SHS)	Liquigen *(SHS)	MCT oil (Cow and Gate) *(SHS)	Duocal *(SHS) per 100 g	Liquid Duocal *(SHS)
Major Ingredients			Peanut oil and water emulsion	Emulsion of medium chain triglycerides and water mainly C_8 and C_{10}	Medium chain triglycerides mainly C_8 and C_{10}	Maltodextrin refined vegetable oil and fats	Maltodextrin refined vegetable oils
Protein g	Tr	2	–	–	–	–	–
Fat g	100	48	50	52	98	22	7
Carbohydrate g	–	2	–	–	–	73	24
Energy kcal	899	447	450	400	830	470	150
Na mmol	Tr	1.2	0.9	1.7	–	1.2	<0.9
K mmol	Tr	2.0	0.5	0.7	–	0.1	<0.8

MIXED SUPPLEMENTS Composition per 100 ml

	Cows milk (Domestic)	Complan Plain (Farley) per 100 g	Build-up Natural (Carnation) per 100 g	Build-up vanilla (Carnation) per 38 g sachet	Fortify (Cow and Gate) per 100 g	Fortimel (Cow and Gate)
Major Ingredients		Skimmed milk powder vegetable oil maltodextrin sucrose vits and mins	Skimmed milk powder sucrose glucose lactose vits and mins	Skimmed milk powder sucrose glucose lactose vits and min	Glucose syrup caseinates vegetable oils vits & mins	Modified skimmed milk sucrose corn oil lecithin maltodextrin vits & mins
Protein g	3.3	20	24.4	9.3	19	9.7
Fat g	3.8	16	0.9	0.3	18	2.1
Carbohydrate g	4.7	55	65.5	24.9	57	10.4
Energy kcal	65	444	351	133	455	100
Na mmol	2.1	15	16.2	6.2	16	2.2
K mmol	3.7	21	24	9	16	5.1

DIETARY SUPPLEMENTS *continued*

MIXED SUPPLEMENTS Composition per 100 ml *continued* | | | | BRANCHED CHAIN AMINO-ACID FORMULAE | |

	Fortisip (Cow and Gate)	Fortisip Energy plus (Cow and Gate)	Nutrauxil Sip (KabiVitrum)	Fresubin (Fresenius)	Hepatamine * (SHS) per 100 g	Hepatonutril (Oxford Nutrition) per 98 g sachet
Major Ingredients	Maltodextrin sodium and calcium caseinate corn, palm, coconut oil vits & mins	Maltodextrin corn, palm, coconut oil lecithin sodium and calcium caseinate vits and mins	Maltodextrin sucrose sunflower oil sodium and calcium caseinate soya protein MCT vits and mins	Milk and soya protein sunflower seed oil oligo and polysaccharide vits & mins	Synthetic amino-acids rich in BCAA low in aromatic amino-acids carbohydrate	Oligopeptides enriched with amino acids 40% BCAA Low in aromatic amino acids polysaccharide MCT oil vits & mins
Protein g	4	5	3.8	3.8	30	12.2
Fat g	4	6.5	3.4	3.4	–	7.2
Carbohydrate g	12	18	13.8	13.8	65	75
Energy kcal	100	150	100	100	345	418
Na mmol	3.5	3.5	3.3	3.3	6.0	4.0
K mmol	3.8	3.8	3.2	3.2	0.6	7.6

COMPOSITION OF INFANT FORMULAE PER 100 ML[a]

| | Whey-based formulae | | | | | Casein based formulae | | | | |
	Mature Breast milk[b]	Cow & Gate Premium[c]	Wyeth SMA Gold Cap[c]	Milupa Aptamil[c]	Farley Osterfeed[c]	Cow & Gate Plus[c]	Wyeth SMA White Cap[c]	Milupa Milumil[c]	Farley Ostermilk Complete Formula[c]	Farley Ostermilk Two[c]
Energy kcal	59	66	65	67	68	66	65	69	65	62
Protein g	1.3	1.5	1.5	1.5	1.45	1.9	1.5	1.9	1.7	1.8
% % Casein: Whey	40:60	40:50	40:60	40:60	40:60	80:20	80:20	80:20	N/A	N/A
Fat g	4.1	3.5	3.6	3.6	3.8	3.4	3.6	3.1	2.6	2.4
CHO g	7.2	7.3	7.2	7.2	7.0	7.3	7.2	8.4	8.6	8.3
MINERALS										
Na mmol	0.6	0.8	0.7	0.8	0.8	1.1	0.9	1.0	1.1	1.1
K mmol	1.5	1.6	1.4	2.1	1.4	2.5	1.9	2.1	1.7	2.0
Cl mmol	1.2	1.1	1.1	1.1	1.26	1.7	1.3	1.2	1.6	1.6
Fe μmol	1.3	9.0	12.1	12.6	11.7	9.0	12.1	7.2	11.7	11.7
Ca mmol	0.9	1.2	1.1	1.5	0.9	2.1	1.4	1.8	1.5	1.6
P mmol	0.5	0.9	1.1	1.1	0.9	1.8	1.4	1.8	1.6	1.7
Mg mmol	0.1	0.2	0.2	0.3	0.2	0.3	0.2	0.3	0.2	0.3
Mn μmol	N/A	0.1	0.3	0.1	0.06	0.1	0.3	0.2	0.06	0.06
Cu μmol	0.6	0.6	0.8	0.7	0.6	0.6	0.8	0.4	0.6	0.6
Zn μmol	4.2	6.0	7.5	6.0	5.3	6.0	7.5	6.0	4.9	4.6
I μmol	N/A	0.05	0.05	0.03	0.04	0.05	0.03	0.02	0.08	0.09
Vitamins										
A μg	60.0	80.0	79.0	69.0	100.0	80.0	79.0	65.0	97.0	95.0
D₃ μg	0.025	1.1	1.05	1.0	1.0	1.1	1.05	1.0	1.0	1.0

	Whey-based formulae					Casein based formulae				
	Mature Breast milk[b]	Cow & Gate Premium[c]	Wyeth SMA Gold Cap[c]	Milupa Aptamil[c]	Farley Osterfeed[c]	Cow & Gate Plus[c]	Wyeth SMA White Cap[c]	Milupa Milumil[c]	Farley Ostermilk Complete Formula[c]	Farley Ostermilk Two[c]
E mg	0.34	1.1	0.95	0.7	0.5	1.1	0.95	0.8	0.46	0.45
K μg	N/A	5.0	5.8	4.0	2.7	5.0	5.8	4.0	2.6	1.5
B$_1$ mg	0.02	0.04	0.08	0.04	0.04	0.04	0.08	0.032	0.04	0.04
B$_2$ mg	0.03	0.1	0.11	0.05	0.05	0.1	0.11	0.049	0.05	0.05
B$_6$ mg	0.01	0.04	0.05	0.03	0.03	0.04	0.05	0.04	0.03	0.03
B$_{12}$ μg	Tr.	0.2	0.11	0.15	0.14	0.2	0.11	0.21	0.13	0.13
Nicotinic Acid mg	0.22	0.4	1.0	0.4	0.7	0.4	1.0	0.24	0.65	0.64
Pantothenic Acid mg	0.25	0.3	0.21	0.4	0.23	0.3	0.21	0.24	0.22	0.22
Biotin μg	0.7	1.5	1.5	1.1	1.0	1.5	1.5	1.1	0.97	0.95
Folic Acid μg	5.0	10.0	5.3	10.0	3.4	10.0	5.3	5.0	3.2	3.1
Mesoinositol mg	N/A	N/A	N/A	N/A	N/A	N/A	N/A	N/A	N/A	N/A
Choline mg	N/A	7.0	N/A	N/A	N/A	7.0	N/A	N/A	N/A	N/A
Vitamin C mg	3.7	8.0	5.8	6.0	6.9	8.0	5.8	7.5	6.4	6.2
Renal Solute Load mOsm/l	86[a]	96	92.1	101	N/A	130	100.8	121	N/A	N/A
Osmolality mOsm/kg	N/A	290	N/A	270	N/A	310	N/A	260	N/A	N/A

a   Manufacturers' data 1986
b   McCance and Widdowson 1978
c   All formulae are available ready to feed or as a powder which is reconstituted by mixing one level scoop into a fluid oz (30 ml) water
d   DHSS Report on Health and Social Subjects 1977, No. 12. The Composition of Mature Human Milk, HMSO, London
N/A   Data unavailable

COMPOSITION OF MODIFIED INFANT FORMULAE PER 100 ML.
(A) SOYA BASED

	Formula S[ab] Soya Food (Cow & Gate)	Wysoy[a] (Wyeth)	Prosobee[ab] (Mead Johnson)	Isomil[a] Soy Protein Infant Formula (Abbott)
Energy kcal	67	67	65	68
Protein g	1.8	2.1	2.0	1.8
	Soy-protein isolate supplemented with L-methionine	Soy-protein isolate supplemented with L-methionine	Soy-protein isolate supplemented with L-methionine	Soy-protein isolate supplemented with L-methionine
Carbohydrate g	6.7	6.9	6.6	6.9
	Glucose syrup (derived from hydrolysis of maize starch)	Corn syrup solids Sucrose	Glucose syrup solids	Corn syrup solids Sucrose
Fat g	3.6	3.6	3.6	3.69
	Mixture of palm, coconut, maize and saffflower oils	Blend of oleic and soy oils, oleo oil (destearinated beef fat) and coconut oil	Corn oil Coconut oil	Corn oil, coconut oil, linoleic acid = 17% total calories
Minerals				
Na mmol	0.8	0.9	1.1	1.4
K mmol	1.6	1.9	1.5	1.9
Cl mmol	1.1	1.1	1.1	1.7

	Formula S[ab] Soya Food (Cow & Gate)	Wysoy[a] (Wyeth)	Prosobee[ab] (Mead Johnson)	Isomil[a] Soy Protein Infant Formula (Abbott)
Fe μmol	9.0	12.0	21.5	21.6
Ca mmol	1.4	1.6	1.4	1.8
P mmol	0.9	1.4	1.3	1.6
Mg mmol	0.2	0.3	0.3	0.2
Mn μmol	0.6	0.4	0.4	0.4
Cu μmol	0.6	0.8	0.9	0.8
Zn μmol	6.0	7.5	7.7	7.5
I μmol	0.1	0.08	0.04	0.08
Molybdenum μmol	N/A	N/A	N/A	N/A
Selenium μmol	N/A	N/A	N/A	N/A
Chromium μmol	N/A	N/A	N/A	N/A
Vitamins				
A μg	80	79	50	60
D_3 μg	1.1	1.05	1.05	1.0
E mg	1.3	0.95	1.5	1.7
K μg	5.0	10.5	10.0	10.0
B_1 mg	0.04	0.08	0.05	0.04
B_2 mg	0.1	0.11	0.06	0.06
B_6 mg	0.04	0.05	0.04	0.04
B_{12} μg	0.2	0.21	0.2	0.3
Nicotinic Acid mg	0.4	1.0	0.8	0.9
Pantothenic Acid mg	0.3	0.32	0.3	0.5
Biotin μg	1.5	3.7	5.0	3.0
Folic acid μg	10.0	5.3	10.0	10.0

Mesoinositol mg	3.5	N/A	N/A	N/A
Choline mg	7.0	9.0	8.5	7.0
Vitamin C mg	8.0	5.8	5.4	5.5
Miscellaneous Renal Solute load mosmol/litre	108	122.4	N/A	122.2
Osmolality mosmol/Kg of H_2O	165	260	160	250
Additional composition information	N/A	Has added: taurine 3.76 mg/100 ml carnitine 0.81 mg/100 ml	N/A	Has added: taurine 4.5 mg/100 ml carnitine 1.18 mg/100 ml
Mixing	1 level scoop (approx. 4.3 g Powder) to 30 ml (1 fluid oz) water	1 level scoop (approx. 4.25 g Powder) to 28 ml (1 fluid oz) water	1 level scoop (approx. 4.3 g Powder) to 30 ml (1 fluid oz) water	1 level scoop to 30 ml (1 fluid oz) water
Recommended dosage	N/A	N/A	N/A	N/A
Indications	Cows' Milk Intolerance Galactosaemia Galactokinase deficiency Lactose intolerance	Cows' Milk Intolerance Lactose Intolerance Galactosaemia Galactokinase deficiency	Cows' milk allergy or intolerance Lactose intolerance Galactosaemia	Cows' Milk Intolerance Lactose Intolerance Galactosaemia Galactokinase deficiency

a lactose and gluten free
b sucrose free

COMPOSITION OF MODIFIED INFANT FORMULAE PER 100 ML.
(B) DEFINED FORMULAE

	Nutramigen (Mead Johnson)	Pregestimil[ab] (Mead Johnson)	Pepdite 0-2[ab] (Scientific Hospital Supplied Ltd)	MCT Pepdite 0-2[ab] (Scientific Hospital Supplies Ltd)	Neocate[ab] (Scientific Hospital Supplies Ltd)
Energy kcal	65	66	70	67	71
Protein g	1.9 Enzymatically-hydrolysed casein.	1.9 Enzymatically-hydrolysed casein supplemented with 1-Tyrosine, 1-Cystine 1-Tryptophan	2.1 Peptides from hydrolysed non-milk protein (soya)	2.1 Peptides from hydrolysed non-milk protein (soya)	2.02 Amino acids
Carbohydrate g	9.1 Sucrose Modified tapioca starch	9.1 Glucose syrup solids Modified tapioca starch	8.4 Maltodextrin	9.4 Maltodextrin	8.4 Maltodextrin
Fat g	2.6 Corn Oil	2.7 Corn oil MCT oil Lecithin	3.5 Coconut fat Ground nut oil Animal fat	2.8 (82% MCT) Fractionated coconut oil Linoleic acid	3.5 Coconut fat Ground nut oil Animal fats
Minerals					
Na mmol	1.3	1.4	1.3	1.9	0.8
K mmol	1.8	1.9	1.5	1.5	1.5

Cl mmol	1.6	1.6	1.1	1.1	1.2
Fe μmol	23.4	23.4	14.4	14.4	14.4
Ca mmol	1.6	1.6	1.1	1.1	1.1
P mmol	1.3	1.3	1.1	1.1	1.1
Mg mmol	0.3	0.3	0.2	0.2	0.2
Mn μmol	0.4	0.4	1.1	1.1	1.1
Cu μmol	0.9	0.9	0.9	0.9	0.9
Zn μmol	6.3	6.3	9.0	9.0	9.0
I μmol	0.04	0.04	0.05	0.05	0.05
Molybdenum μmol	N/A	N/A	0.04	0.04	0.04
Selenium μmol	N/A	N/A	0.03	0.03	0.03
Chromium μmol	N/A	N/A	0.04	0.04	0.04
Vitamins					
A μg	51	63	80.0	80.0	80.0
D_3 μg	0.3	1.1	1.1	1.1	1.1
E mg	1.1	1.6	0.7	0.7	0.7
K μg	10.5	11.0	6.8	6.8	6.8
B_1 mg	0.35	0.05	0.05	0.06	0.06
B_2 mg	0.36	0.06	0.03	0.09	0.09
B_6 mg	0.04	0.04	0.05	0.05	0.05
B_{12} μg	0.2	0.21	0.15	0.15	0.15
Nicotinic Acid mg	0.35	0.85	0.7	0.7	0.7
Pantothenic Acid mg	0.32	0.32	0.25	0.25	0.25
Biotin μg	5.3	0.005	3.9	3.9	3.9
Folic acid μg	10.5	10.6	5.8	5.8	5.8
Mesoinositol mg	3.3	3.2	15.0	15.0	15.0
Choline mg	9.0	9.0	9.8	9.8	9.8
Vitamin C mg	5.5	5.5	6.2	6.2	6.2
Osmolality mosmol/Kg of H_2O	320	338	195	337	320

	Nutramigen (Mead Johnson)	Pregestimil[ab] (Mead Johnson)	Pepdite 0–2[ab] (Scientific Hospital Supplied Ltd)	MCT Pepdite 0–2[ab] (Scientific Hospital Supplies Ltd)	Neocate[ab] (Scientific Hospital Supplies Ltd)
Mixing	1 level scoop (4.9 g powder) to 30 ml (2 fluid oz) water	1 level scoop (4.9 g powder) to 30 ml (1 fluid oz) water	1 level scoop (approx 5 g) to 30 ml (1 fluid oz) water	1 level scoop (approx 5 g) to 30 ml (1 fluid oz) water	1 level scoop (5 g powder) to 30 ml (1 fluid oz) water
Manufacturers' recommended dosage	Only suitable for infants over 3 months	N/A	25 g/Kg body weight/day	25 g/Kg body weight/day	25 g/Kg body weight/day
Indications	Lactose intolerance Galactosaemia Sensitivity to milk and other whole proteins. Persistant diarrhoea of infectious origin	Lactose and/or sucrose intolerance Sensitivity to intact protein Intractable diarrhoea Idiopathic defects of digestion or absorption Fat malabsorption Multiple nutrient malabsorption states following intestinal resection	Milk protein or other whole protein intolerance Feeding difficulties in post operative conditions Intractable malabsorption Chronic intestinal disease Short bowel syndrome Galactosaemia Lactose intolerance	Milk protein or other whole protein intolerance Feeding difficulties in post operative conditions Intractable malabsorption Chronic intestinal disease Short bowel syndrome Cystic Fibrosis Lymphatic disorders	Milk proteir or other whole protein intolerance Feeding difficulties in post operative conditions Intractable malabsorption Chronic intestinal disease Short bowel syndrome Galactosaemia Lactose intolerance

a   lactose and gluten free
b   sucrose free
Manufacturers' data 1986.

CALORIE AND PROTEIN VALUES OF COMMON FOODS

Bread, cereals, biscuits, cakes

	kcal	Protein g
1 slice bread, large loaf (40 g)	90	3.5
2 cream crackers	70	1.5
2 crispbreads	50	1.5
2 semi-sweet biscuits, e.g. Rich Tea	70	1.0
2 sweet biscuits	100	1.0
Small bowl of breakfast cereal (20 g)	70	1.5
Small bowl of porridge made with water (120 g)	60	1.5
Boiled rice, 1 tablespoon (40 g)	50	1.0
Boiled macaroni or other pasta, 1 tablespoon (40 g)	50	1.5
Shortcrust pastry, 1 small square (20 g)	100	1.0
Currant bun (50 g)	150	3.5
Jam tart (40 g)	150	1.5
Fruit Cake, small slice (60 g)	200	2.0
Custard tart, individual (70 g)	200	4.0
Victoria sandwich, 1 slice (60 g)	180	2.0
Jam doughnut (70 g)	238	4.0

Meat, fish, eggs, milk, cheese

2 rashers fried bacon (30 g)	140	7
Roast meat or poultry, 2 thin slices (60 g)	120	15
Stewed beef, 1 tablespoon (40 g)	50	4
Steak and kidney pie, an individual (100 g)	320	9
1 grilled large sausage (40 g)	125	5
Individual pork pie (120 g)	450	12
Grilled fish, 1 small fillet (90 g)	80	18
Fried battered fish, 1 small fillet (100 g)	200	20
Fish fingers, 3 fried	150	8
Eggs, 1 boiled or poached	75	6
1 scrambled or omelette	120	8
1 fried	115	7
Milk, 1 glass, ⅓ pint	130	7
Yoghurt, natural, 1 small carton	75	7
fruit, 1 small carton	150	7
Cheese, Cheddar, matchbox size piece (40 g)	160	10
Edam, matchbox size piece (40 g)	120	10
Stilton, matchbox size piece (40 g)	185	10
Cottage, 1 small tub (120 g)	110	16

CALORIE AND PROTEIN VALUES OF COMMON FOODS *Continued*

Fats and sugars

	kcal	Protein g
Butter or margarine, individual portion (8 g)	60	—
Cream, single, 1 tablespoon (20 ml)	45	0.5
double, 1 tablespoon (20 ml)	90	—
Mayonnaise, 1 tablespoon (30 g)	200	0.5
Sugar, 1 teaspoon (5 g)	20	—
Jam, honey, marmalade, syrup, 1 teaspoon (15 g)	40	—
Chocolate, 2 squares (15 g)	75	1.0
Boiled sweets (8 g)	25	—
Mars bar (60 g)	270	3.0

Vegetables and fruit

Most vegetables and salad ingredients contribute a small amount to overall calorie protein intake but are a valuable source of vitamins, minerals and fibre.

	kcal	Protein g
1 small potato, boiled/jacket (50 g)	45	0.5
1 small potato, roast (50 g)	75	1.5
Chips, 1 tablespoon (40 g)	100	2.0
Potato crisps, 1 small packet	135	1.5
Baked beans in tomato sauce, 2 tablespoons (80 g)	70	5.0
1 medium apple/orange/pear/peach/banana	50	—
Sultans, currants, raisins, 1 tablespoon (15 g)	40	—
Handful of grapes (75 g)	50	—
Bowlful of strawberries or raspberries (175 g)	40	—

Puddings

	kcal	Protein g
Rice pudding, small bowl (120 g)	120	4.0
Sponge pudding, small bowl (90 g)	300	5.0
Stewed fruit + sugar or tinned fruit, small bowl (100 g)	80	0.5
Fruit pie, 1 slice (90 g)	150	2.0
Evaporated milk, 1 tablespoon (20 ml)	30	1.5
Custard, 1 tablespoon (20 ml)	25	1.0
Ice cream, 1 brickette (40 g)	65	1.0

Snacks

	kcal	Protein g
Bowl of tinned soup (200 ml)	100	3.0
Cheese roll or 2 cream crackers + butter and cheese portion	220	8.0
Small packet peanuts (25 g)	140	6.0
Sausage roll, small (30 g)	140	3.0
1 round ham sandwiches	240	10.0
Chocolate biscuit, full coated (25 g)	130	1.5

Drinks

	kcal	Protein g
Cup of tea or coffee, milk no sugar	20	1.0
Cup of chocolate, Ovaltine or Horlicks, all milk	130	6.0
Glass of milk (200 ml)	130	7.0
Glass of natural orange juice (200 ml)	66	–
Glass of diluted orange squash (200 ml)	40	–
Glass of Coca-Cola or other fizzy drink (200 ml)	80	–
½ pint beer (250 ml)	75	0.5
1 glass of wine (150 ml)	100	–
1 tot of spirit, 1/0 gill (20 ml)	45	–

MANUFACTURERS ADDRESSES

United Kingdom

Abbott Laboratories Ltd
Queenborough
Kent, ME11 5EL
(0795) 663371

Allen & Hanburys Ltd
Horsenden House
Oldfield Lane North
Greenford
Middlesex UB6 0HB
(01) 422 4225

Argyle
Division of Sherwood Medical
London Road
Crawley
West Sussex RH10 2 TL
(0293) 34501

Avon Medical Ltd
Moon Boat Drive
Redditch
Worcs, B98 9HA
(0527) 64901

Beecham Research Laboratories
Brentford
Middlesex TW8 9BD
(01) 560 5151

Bencard
(see Beecham)

Boots Company Ltd
Thane Road
Nottingham, NG2 3AA
(0602) 506255

B Braun Medical Ltd
Evett Close
Stocklake
Aylesbury, Bucks, HP20 1DN
(0296) 432626

Bristol-Myers Co Ld
Swakeleys House
Milton Road
Ickenham
Uxbridge UB10 8NS
(08956) 39911

Carnation Health Care
36 Park Street
Croydon
Surrey CR9 1TT
(01) 686-3333

Cow and Gate Ltd
Trowbridge
Wilts, BA14 9HZ
(02214) 68381

Duncan, Flockhart & Co Ltd
700 Oldfield Lane North, Greenford
Middlesex UB6 0HD
(01) 422 2331

Evans Medical Ltd
318 High Street North
Dunstable
Beds LU6 1BE
(0582) 608308

Farley Health Products
P.O. Box 94
Thane Road West
Nottingham
NG2 3AA
(0602) 592 389

Fresenius Dylade
50 Brindley Road
Astmoor Industrial Estate
Runcorn
Cheshire WA7 1PG
(09285) 65011

Geistlich Sons Ltd
Newton Bank
Long Lane
Chester, CH2 3QZ
(0244) 47534

Glaxo Laboratories Ltd
891–995 Greenford Road
Greenford
Middlesex, UB6 0HE
(01) 422 3434

IMED Ltd
Milton Trading Estate
Abingdon
Oxon, OX14 4RX
(0235) 83211

International Medication Systems
  (UK) Ltd
11 Royal Oak Way South
Daventry
Northamptonshire NN11 5PJ
(0327) 703231

KabiVitrum Ltd
Riverside Way
Uxbridge
Middlesex UB8 2YF
(0895) 51144

Leo Laboratories Ltd
Longwick Road
Princes Risborough
Bucks HP17 9RR
(084 44) 7333

Macarthy's Surgical Ltd
Selinas Lane
Dagenham RM8 1QD
(01) 593 7511

Mead Johnson Nutritionals
(see Bristol-Myers Co Ltd)

Merck E Ltd
Winchester Road
Four Marts
Alton, Hants GU34 5HG
(0420) 64011

Miramed; Agents:-
Oxford Nutrition Ltd
P.O. Box 31
Oxford OX2 8H3
(0865) 58045

Norwich Eaton Ltd
Hedley House
St Nicholas Ave
Gosforth
Newcastle NE3 1LR
(091) 279 2100

Paines and Byrne Ltd
Bilton Road
Perivale
Greenford
Middlesex UB6 7HG
(01) 997 1143

Parke-Davis & Co Ltd
Mitchell House
Southampton Road
Eastleigh, Hants SO5 5RY
(0703) 619791

Pfrimmer Viggo
(U.K. agent: see Merck)

Pharmacia Ltd
Hospital Products
Pharmacia House
Midsummer Boulevard
Milton Keynes MK9 3HP
(0908) 661101

Portex Ltd
Hythe
Kent, CT21 6JL
(0303) 66863

MANUFACTURERS ADDRESSES *continued*

Roussel Laboratories Ltd
Broadwater Park
North Orbital Road
Uxbridge
Middlesex UB9 5HP
(0895) 834343

Scientific Hospital Supplies Ltd
38 Queensland Street
Liverpool, L7 3JG
(051) 708 8008

Schuco International London Ltd
Woodhouse Road
London NI2 0NE
(01) 368 1642

Searle Pharmaceuticals Ltd
P.O. Box 53
Lane End Road
High Wycombe
Bucks, HP12 4HL
(0494) 21124

Travenol Laboratories Ltd
Thorpe Lea Road
Egham
Surrey TW20 8HY
(0784) 34388

Unigreg Ltd
15/17 Worple Road
Wimbledon
London, SW19 4JS
(01) 946 7745

Viomedex Ltd
Gordon Road
Buxted
Uckfield
East Sussex, TN22 4LH
(082581) 3566

Vygon (UK) Ltd
Bridge Road
Cirencester
Gloucestershire
GL7 1PT
(0285) 67051/2/3

Wyeth Laboratories
Huntercombe Lane South
Taplow
Maidenhead
Berks SL6 0PH
(06286) 4377

North America

Abbott Laboratories Ltd
Ross Laboratories
625 Cleveland Avenue
Columbus, Ohio 43216

Argyle
Argyle Division
Sherwood Medical Industries Inc
1831 Olive Street
St Louis 3
Missouri 63103

Beecham
Beecham Laboratories
501 Fifth Street
Bristol, Tennessee 37620

Beecham Inc
Western Hemisphere Division
65 Industrial South
Clifton, New Jersey 07012

Carnation
Carnation International
5045 Wilshire Boulevard
Los Angeles
California 90036

Glaxo
Glaxo Latin America Inc
Suite 608
The International Building
2455 East Sunrise Boulevard
Fort Lauderdale
Florida 33304

Glaxo Canada Ltd
1025 The Queensway
Toronto
Ontario, M8Z 556

IMED
IMED Corporation
9925 Carroll Canyon Road
San Diego
California 92131

IMED Canada Ltd
6535 Millcreek Drive
Unit 11, Mississanga
Ontario, L5N 2M2

KabiVitrum
Cutler International
2200 Powell Street
Emeryville
California 94608

Pharmacia (Canada) Ltd
2044 St Regis Blvd
Dorval, Quebec H9P 1H6

Mead Johnson
Bristol-Myers Company
International Division
2404 Pennsylvania Avenue
Evansville
Indiana 47721

Norwich Eaton
Norwich-Eaton Pharmaceuticals
PO Box 191
Norwich, New York 13815

Paines & Byrne
Supplied from
United Kingdom

Parke-Davis
Warner-Lambert
201 Tabor Road
PO Box 377
Morris Plains
New Jersey 07950

Roussel
Roussel (Canada) Ltd
4045 Cote Vertu
Montreal
Quebec H4R 2E8

Searle
G.D. Searle International Co
PO Box 1045
Skokie, Illinois 60076

Australia

Argyle
Argyle Division
Sherwood Medical Industries (Pty)
Ltd
84–86 Dalmeny Avenue
Rosebery NSW 2018

Beecham
Beecham Research Laboratories
6–9 Winterton Road
PO Box 59
Clayton, Victoria 3168

Carnation
Carnation Company (Pty) Ltd
612–616 St Kilda Road
Melbourne
Victoria 3004

MANUFACTURERS ADDRESSES *continued*

Glaxo
 Glaxo Australia Pty Ltd
 PO Box 168
 Boronia
 Victoria V155

IMED
 IMED Australia Pty Ltd
 1 Clyde Street
 Rydal More
 New South Wales 2116

KabiVitrum
 Pharmacia (South Seas) Pty Ltd
 4 Byfield Street
 PO Box 175
 North Ryde
 New South Wales 2112

 Tuta Laboratories
  (Australia) Pty Ltd
 PO Box 166
 Lane Cove
 New South Wales 2066

Mead Johnson
 Bristol-Myers Company Pty Ltd
 345 Pacific Highway
 Crows Nest
 New South Wales 2065

Norwich Eaton
 Norwich Eaton Pty Ltd
 Lombard House
 781 Pacific Highway
 Chatswood
 New South Wales 2067

Paines & Byrne
 A.E. Stanson & Co Pty Ltd
 PO Box 118
 Mount Waverley
 Victoria 3149

Parke-Davis
 Warner-Lambert Pty
 PO Box 327
 North Sydney
 New South Wales 2060

Roussel
 Roussel Pharmaceuticals Pty Ltd
 Gladstone Road
 PO Box 193
 Castle Hill
 New South Wales 2134

Searle
 G.D. Searle (Australia) Pty Ltd
 9th Floor, Mainline Building
 8 West Street, North Sydney
 New South Wales 2060

Vygon
 A.E. Stansen & Co
 PO Box 118
 Mount Waverley
 Victoria 3149

Index